Australian & New Zealand Edition

Beating Sugar Addiction

FOR

DUMMIES®

A Wiley Brand

T0324372

Australian & New Zealand Edition

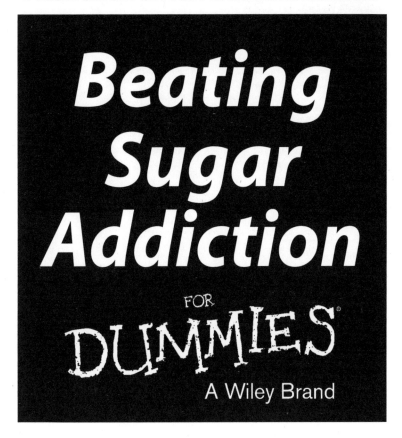

Beating Sugar Addiction

FOR

DUMMIES

A Wiley Brand

by Michele Chevalley Hedge
Dan DeFigio

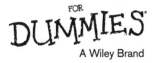

FOR
DUMMIES
A Wiley Brand

Beating Sugar Addiction For Dummies®, Australian & New Zealand Edition

Published by
Wiley Publishing Australia Pty Ltd
42 McDougall Street
Milton, Qld 4064
www.dummies.com

Copyright © 2014 Wiley Publishing Australia Pty Ltd

Authorised adaptation of *Beating Sugar Addiction For Dummies* (ISBN 9781118546451)

The moral rights of the authors have been asserted

National Library of Australia
Cataloguing-in-Publication data:

Author:	Chevalley Hedge, Michele
Title:	Beating Sugar Addiction For Dummies / Michele Chevalley Hedge, Dan DeFigio.
Edition:	Australian and New Zealand ed.
ISBN:	9781118641187 (pbk.)
	9781118641217 (ebook)
Series:	For Dummies
Notes:	Includes index.
Subjects:	Sugar — Health aspects
	Sugar-free diet
Other authors/ contributors:	DeFigio, Dan.
Dewey Number:	641.336

Cover image: © Hugh Threlfall/Getty Images

Typeset by diacriTech, Chennai, India

Printed in Singapore by
C.O.S. Printers Pte Ltd

10 9 8 7 6 5 4 3 2 1

Contents at a Glance

Recipes at a Glance

Table of Contents

Introduction

A high-sugar diet is one of the primary causes of obesity, diabetes, depression, stress and anxiety issues, and a host of other health problems. Sadly, a quick look at current health-care statistics indicates that these 'lifestyle' diseases are on a parallel rise across the board with the increase in sugar consumption. Chances are, you know people who have a health-related illness that can be traced back to poor nutrition — or perhaps you're in danger of such an illness yourself. High blood pressure, high cholesterol, digestive issues and cardiovascular problems are just a few of the illnesses discussed daily.

We have both had the pleasure of changing the lives of thousands of people just through changing the simple act of eating! We have witnessed firsthand how sugar abuse is addictive, and physically, mentally and emotionally destabilising. We've seen people from all walks of life and many different backgrounds — otherwise smart and capable individuals completely defeated by poor nutrition — begin to flourish on a low-sugar, whole-foods way of life.

Sugar is just as addictive as cocaine, but it's cheap, legal and socially acceptable. If people were selling a drug that had the same damaging effects as sugar, the government would insist they stop selling it immediately. Yet, sugar is everywhere — in cereals, soft drinks, sport drinks, burger buns, peanut butter, and even in flavoured milks. Sugar addiction and other unhealthy lifestyle habits stem from (and result in) poor nutrition, lack of sleep and stress. It's our hope that this book reaches many more people than we could possibly help in nutrition consultation, and serves as a motivating guidebook and a beacon of hope for the millions of people struggling with sugar addiction, weight gain, stress, diabetes, exhaustion, poor self-esteem and depression.

About This Book

Beating sugar addiction requires more than just staying away from sweet treats. To truly transition into a new healthy lifestyle, you must look into the motivation behind your behaviour, figure out what emotional holes you've been trying to fill with sugar, and understand how you're going to create this new lifestyle so it becomes habitual and easy for you to sustain.

We wrote this book with the intention of leading you through the process of getting off sugar, feeling good about yourself, and living a healthier lifestyle. As you go through the process, you'll find that it may also help you investigate, understand, and ultimately change your behaviour and mindset about lots of things — this is about much more than just cutting out sugar! When you begin to feel good physically and mentally, you feel better about most things in your life.

Herein you find chapters about understanding sugar, carbohydrates and the psychology of sugar addiction; navigating restaurants and special occasions; eating mindfully; building a support system; 'cleansing' your pantry; and — most importantly — breaking the cycle of failure and frustration, leading to a low-sugar life that's healthy, empowered and under your own control.

Throughout this book, we use the word *sugar* to mean a low-nutrient, sweet carbohydrate like table sugar, lollies, soft drinks or high-fructose corn syrup, as opposed to the technical definition of a sugar that a chemist would use. Other sources of carbohydrates you digest (like vegetables and grains) are technically broken down into simple sugars too, but we ask the technical wizards to forgive us as we use the word *sugar* in more conventional terms, referring to junk food and processed sweeteners.

Here are some other conventions to keep in mind while digging into this book:

- ✔ We discuss a lot of health issues, but please understand that we refer to medical conditions and diseases in general terms only. You shouldn't consider the advice or information contained in this book to be pertinent to your specific situation — always consult with a qualified medical practitioner or nutrition consultant for more personalised information.

- ✔ We use *italics* for terms that we define or that we want to emphasise. Web addresses appear in `monofont` so they're easy to pick out.

- ✔ Part IV of this book is full of recipes, and in it we use the metric system of measurement, so temperatures are in Celsius, measurements are in cups, millilitres and grams, and so on.

- ✔ In the recipes, do your best to use organic ingredients whenever possible. Eggs should be from pasture-fed, antibiotic-free chickens. Choose fresh fruits, vegetables, grains and herbs that are organic to avoid pesticides and genetically modified ingredients. All meat should ideally be pasture-raised without antibiotics. Buy fish that is wild-caught, not farmed.

- ☙ This tomato icon highlights the vegetarian recipes in the book.

Some chapters contain *sidebars* — sections of text enclosed in boxes that give additional information, more technical details, or bonus advice that's not essential to the main text. If you're pressed for time, feel free to skip over the sidebars and perhaps come back to them later.

You can also jump over the items marked by the Technical Stuff icon. With these discussions, we go a little deeper into the science or technical details of a particular issue.

Foolish Assumptions

While working on this book, we made some general assumptions about who would be reading it:

✔ We assume that you feel busy and overwhelmed on a regular basis, and that you often resort to stress eating or medicating with sugar. And, most importantly, you want to stop doing this!

✔ We assume that you've struggled for a long time with food confusion, losing weight, sticking to healthy eating plans and getting control over your life in general, and you need dietary advice that's both effective and realistic.

✔ We assume that you have lots of things packed into your schedule, and you don't have all day to just sit around and read. We've attempted to be reasonably thorough, without getting too technical or wordy, while delivering valuable information in a concise fashion. You can find additional information and resources online at www.ahealthyview.com.au.

Icons Used in This Book

Throughout the margins of this book you find symbols that spotlight important points, examples and warnings. Look for these icons:

This icon marks information that's important to remember, or may represent a good summary of a larger section. These may be worth reading twice or jotting down if you're a note-taker.

We love knowing the details of how and why things work the way they do, and nutrition science and physiology are not exceptions. Unfortunately for some of you, we also love to explain these details when we write. So if you're not into scientific explanations, feel free to skip the paragraphs marked with this icon.

Tidbits and takeaway messages are marked with this icon. These are nuggets that you may want to highlight or forward to your friends.

The Warning icon cautions you about something potentially harmful. When you see this icon, pay careful attention to the corresponding text.

Beyond the Book

In addition to the material in the print or ebook you're reading right now, *Beating Sugar Addiction For Dummies*, Australian and New Zealand Edition, also comes with some access-anywhere goodies on the internet. Check out the free Cheat Sheet at www.dummies.com/cheatsheet/ beatingsugaraddictionau for some quick, helpful tips. For free extra companion material for this book, visit www.dummies.com/extras/ beatingsugaraddictionau.

Where to Go from Here

You don't have to read *Beating Sugar Addiction For Dummies* from cover to cover before you begin your journey to free yourself from sugar! This book (like all *For Dummies* books) is written in modular fashion, with each chapter pretty much standing on its own. We hope that you read through each chapter eventually (because each one contains a lot of valuable information and food for thought that you may not already know), but you certainly don't have to read this book straight through.

Feel free to look over the table of contents so you can skip around to the topics that interest you most. In each chapter, we often direct you to other sections of the book that expand on a given subject or that give you more tips or information about the topic at hand.

For starters, we suggest that you read through Chapter 1 to get a quick overview of the major topics contained in this book — it's short, but it gives you a taste of everything so you can figure out what you want to read about next.

If you're ready to start making changes right away, move on to Chapter 2, where you can take the quizzes to find out which kind of sugar addict you might resemble and what some of your major motivations and mindsets may be. After you understand the whys of your sugar problem, you can flip to Chapter 9 and start working on your sugar-free lifestyle right away!

If you'd like to find out more about sugar and how it affects your body (including why it's so addictive), spend some time on Chapters 3 and 4. If you feel like working out, Chapter 12 explains how to exercise for maximum results in minimal time.

Do you need help with making better food choices or doing a kitchen makeover? Chapters 5 and 6 are all about nutrition and how to overhaul your pantry, kitchen and refrigerator. When it's time to cook, Part IV contains all the recipes for low-sugar breakfasts, lunches, dinners, snacks and desserts.

If your theme has been, 'I know what I'm supposed to do, but I'm just not doing it', flip to Chapter 8 to read about mindfulness and being intentional instead of reactive.

Whatever you choose to read first, enjoy it — and, more importantly, implement it!

Part I

Are You a Sugar Addict or a Sweet Tooth?

getting started
with
beating
sugar
addiction

In this part . . .

- ✔ Take a quiz to determine what type of sugar addict you might be so that you can start understanding and changing your behaviours.

- ✔ Get to the physical, chemical and emotional roots of why sugar is so addictive.

- ✔ Uncover the truth about carbohydrates and sugars, and sort out good carbs from bad.

- ✔ Recognise some hidden sources of sugar and get the facts about artificial sweeteners.

- ✔ Understand the effect sugar has on your brain as well as its negative effects on your overall health.

Chapter 1

Moving from Sugar Addiction to Sugar Reduction

. . . .

In This Chapter

▶ Explaining the nature of sugar addiction

▶ Taking the first steps of your low-sugar journey

▶ Turning your life around by changing your thinking

. . . .

*I*n small amounts, sugar is an innocuous substance. Every cell in your body needs sugar (glucose) to survive and function, so your digestive system breaks down the carbohydrates you eat into glucose to fuel your body and your brain. A major problem with the modern diet is that sugar is present (and hidden) in *enormous* amounts, instead of in the small amounts found in natural foods. Processed foods, sweetened beverages, engineered sweeteners and refined grains are pervasive in the Western food supply, overloading your body with unmanageable amounts of sugar and chemicals.

We're not exaggerating when we say that sugar is just as addictive as cocaine. It acts on the pleasure centre of the brain just like alcohol and heroin, so the more you eat, the more you want. Combine sugar's addictive nature with its omnipresence in society, and you get a recipe for a global health disaster. Reaching for quick, processed and convenient 'foods' during a stressful, time-poor day is all too easy for people, and eventually they become addicted — both to the sugar and to the crazy lifestyle that leads them to it.

Our goal is to guide you through the steps you need to take, both physically and emotionally, to wean yourself away from relying on sugar. This book should be helpful for not only the sugar addict but also those who may not be truly addicted but who are searching for ways to decrease their reliance on stress eating and processed foods in order to live a healthier lifestyle with greater mental and emotional clarity, and optimal wellness.

As you read this chapter, you'll start to understand the magnitude of the harmful effects that overdosing on sugar has on your physical, mental and emotional health and the reasons why sugar can be so addictive. We share some easy tips to improve your eating without being neurotic or trying to be perfect. (We don't do extremes — they don't work and are often temporary patches.) You will get a chance to start unravelling the psychology of your sugar abuse and start looking at how you can begin to change your life by changing your thinking.

Understanding Sugar Addiction

As a species, humans evolved eating the small amounts of sugar found naturally in fruits and plants. Today, Australians and New Zealanders consume approximately 31 teaspoons of sugar every day. We consume that in both added, hidden sugar and in natural sugar, so most of us don't realise how much sugar we're consuming. More than 75 per cent of most people's sugar consumption comes from processed, manufactured foods and drinks. Your body isn't designed to handle the massive load of sugar that the modern diet thrusts upon you, and Australia and New Zealand shoulder the embarrassing obesity, diabetes and metabolic syndrome statistics to prove it.

If Australians and New Zealanders continue with their current lifestyle, obesity rates will continue to rise. In Australia, health experts estimate that, by 2025, 83 per cent of men and 75 per cent of women over 20 will be overweight or obese. New Zealand continues to have one of the highest rates of obesity in the world, only just behind the United States and Mexico in the developed world.

As people get heavier, rates of type 2 diabetes also increase — by 2031, experts predict 3.3 million Australians will have type 2 diabetes. Mainly due to these increased rates of type 2 diabetes, the number of overweight and obese Australians and New Zealanders will place an enormous burden on the health-care system. At the time of writing, type 2 diabetes costs the Australian community $14.6 billion a year — and this will double to $30 billion in 12 years if preventative measures aren't taken. New Zealand can expect similarly high costs on their health-care system — so much so that New Zealand's Ministry of Health is recognising the fast-growing rates of diabetes as a national priority.

Defining sugar addiction

An *addiction* is anything that you must have to avoid a negative feeling or symptom, or the compulsion to artificially produce a pleasurable sensation. Sugar addicts use sugar as an energy booster (to avoid feeling tired and hungry) and a mood lifter because sugar triggers the production of *serotonin* and *dopamine*, which are hormones that make you feel happy and satisfied.

(Alcohol and cocaine are other addictive substances that trigger serotonin and dopamine production.) As with drugs or other addictive substances, those who abuse sugar develop a tolerance to its effects and need more and more of it to yield the same rewards.

You're probably a sugar addict if two or more of the following descriptions rings true for you:

✔ Without sugar, you suffer extreme fatigue or have trouble concentrating.

✔ You eat sugar compulsively, even though you realise the negative consequences.

✔ You experience physical withdrawal symptoms if you go without sugar for a day or two.

✔ You find yourself obsessing over what your next sugar hit will be and when it will be.

✔ You hide your sugar consumption from other people or lie about your eating behaviour.

✔ You need more and more sugar to experience the 'boost'. Foods that used to taste sweet to you don't seem so sweet anymore.

✔ You repeatedly eat too much sugar, even though you promise yourself that you'll never do it again.

✔ You turn to sugar for an emotional lift, such as when you feel lonely or when you've had a bad day.

In Chapter 2 we categorise four types of stereotypical sugar addicts: the Exhausted Addict, the Sad Eater, the Numb Eater and the Sugar Stalker. Head to Chapter 2 and take the quizzes provided to find out what kind of sugar addict (or which combination of addicts) you are so you can regain optimal health and lower your sugar consumption.

Realising how harmful sugar can be

We're not saying you can never have sugar again — what we advocate is that you need to be aware of what sugars you're eating and realise how harmful sugar is to your overall wellbeing. Sugar is an addictive substance and a driving force (or at least an aggravating factor) behind obesity, diabetes, liver disease, autoimmune disorders, chronic fatigue, depression, mood swings, high cholesterol, osteoporosis, cancer, polycystic ovarian syndrome (PCOS), insulin resistance, digestive issues and metabolic syndrome.

These days the damaging diet begins in childhood and, as a result, young people are experiencing the devastating conditions and illnesses formerly reserved for the ageing. Childhood obesity and diabetes are at an all-time high, leading most experts to believe that young people will have major problems much earlier in life because of their junk food diet. Despite popular thinking, childhood weight gain isn't just 'puppy fat' that will reduce as the child ages — obese and overweight children are often likely to stay that way into adulthood. Shockingly, these health issues mean children today are part of a generation that may have a shorter lifespan, by up to ten years, than their own parents.

Weighing the global ramifications of sugar

Because overconsumption of sugar causes so many health problems, it places an enormous burden on an already struggling health-care system (see Chapter 4 for more info on the health hazards of sugar and its consequences on the health-care system). Here are some examples:

- **Shocking obesity statistics:** Statistically, *not* being overweight is unusual in Australia and New Zealand! According to the Australian Bureau of Statistics (ABS), in 2012, 70 per cent of men and 56 per cent of women were overweight or obese, while 25 per cent of children were overweight or obese. In New Zealand, obesity rates are soaring, with the country's population the third most obese in the developed world, only behind the United States and Mexico. Of New Zealand's children, 10 per cent are already obese by the age of 14!

- **Diabetes woes:** Diabetes Australia reports that 280 Australians develop diabetes every day and it is our fastest growing chronic disease. At the time of writing, nearly one million Australians are currently diagnosed with diabetes. However, for each person diagnosed, another one person is not, making the more likely total of Australians with diabetes closer to 1.7 million. Alarmingly, the total number of people with diabetes and pre-diabetes is estimated at 3.2 million. Figures in New Zealand are similar. With current trends, diabetes will become the number one disease in Australia and New Zealand in the next five years. According to Diabetes Australia, the good news is that up to 60 per cent of the cases of type 2 diabetes can be prevented.

- **Healthcare costs crisis:** Obesity and the associated health problems that go along with it place a significant economic burden on the Australian and New Zealand health-care systems. The National Health Medicine Research Council of Australia estimates the direct costs of diabetes in Australia to be between $8 and $21 billion, with the total direct, indirect and social costs estimated at being between $37.7 and $56.6 billion. By 2023, the council predicts the health expenditure for type 2 diabetes will have risen from $1.4 billion to $7 billion per year. Similar health-care expenditure increases are expected in New Zealand.

Strategies that help lower the prevalence of obesity and type 2 diabetes in Australia and New Zealand will not only benefit the health system but also, equally importantly, improve productivity in the workplace, and help ensure better wellbeing and quality of life. With the consistent rise in the rates of obesity and diabetes in the developed world (along with the concomitant rise in related diseases and conditions), the cost of treating these 'lifestyle diseases' will take a bigger and bigger chunk of your pay cheque, until good nutrition and regular exercise become normal instead of 'health nut' behaviour.

One of the most dangerous and seldom-discussed effects of a high-sugar diet is *tissue glycation*. Sugar causes a harmful chemical reaction in the tissues, forming molecules called *advanced glycation end products* (AGEs) that make your tissues stiffer and less elastic. Ironically, these AGEs lead to ageing! The more sugar you eat, the more AGEs you develop, and these damaging molecules cause wrinkles, cataracts, stiff muscles, vascular disease, and brain damage. Recent studies have tied brain dysfunction directly to excess sugar consumption, with healthy insulin levels shown to be crucial for memory and learning. These studies are leading researchers to investigate the connection between sugar consumption and Alzheimer's and dementia.

Getting Off Sugar without Driving Yourself Crazy

Despite what you may believe, getting off sugar and eating a healthier diet don't require superhuman discipline, some infomercial's 'secret' pills, or a lifetime dedicated to eating like a rabbit. Try these easy steps to begin your journey, and consult Chapter 9 for more details:

- ✔ **Keep sugar and junk food out of your house.** You can't eat what you don't have! Remove the obvious culprits like soft drink, lollies, brownies, cake and pastries; also get rid of fruit juice, white-flour products, dried fruit, energy drinks, and anything with the word *syrup* or *sugar* in the first five ingredients. See Chapter 3 for more information about carbohydrates and hidden sources of sugar that you may not be aware of, and consult Chapter 6 for tips on how to do a successful pantry cleanse.

- ✔ **Eat enough during the day.** Eating a combination of protein, quality fats and some complex carbohydrates (preferably from vegetables) every few hours helps keep your blood sugar levels stable and prevents your appetite from getting out of control. When blood sugar levels drop too low, you become ravenously hungry, and you're more likely to grab whatever convenience food is handy. Not eating enough during the day is one of the primary causes of overeating at night, which contributes to weight gain and late-night cravings. Turn to Chapter 5 for a lesson in putting together healthy combinations of protein and carbs throughout the day.

- ✔ **Get enough sleep.** Lack of sleep, stress and sugar cravings create a vicious circle of frustration and fatigue. Stress keeps you up at night, so during the day you walk around exhausted, which increases your desire to use sugar as a convenient pick-me-up. High sugar consumption creates an inflammatory response in your body that creates more physical stress. Some studies suggest that healthy 18-year-olds who undergo sleep deprivation for a few weeks can unfortunately alter their metabolic profile to look like that of a 65-year-old. Reducing your dependence on sugar does much more than just help you sleep better; visit Chapter 7 to find out additional ways that a sugar detox can benefit you.

✔ **Stop eating fat-free.** You may still be conditioned from the 1990s to think that fat-free versions of foods are healthier than their natural counterparts, but the equation consists of more than just counting fat grams. Food manufacturers like to persuade the public with marketing terms like 'fat-free' or 'low-fat', but these foods typically have more sugar or artificial ingredients to make up for the missing fat. One kilogram of sugar is still fat-free on a label. Small amounts of good quality fats in your diet provide tastiness and a feeling of fullness — and these good quality fats will *not* make you fat.

✔ **When you go out to eat at restaurants or special events, don't arrive hungry.** Restaurants are notorious for serving up large portions with hidden-sugar sauces, and for presenting a tantalising dessert menu to boot. Special events like parties and receptions are often sugar-fests, with dead food (food that is low in nutritional value) and alcohol served as far as the eye can see. To help you make sensible choices while you're out, eat a handful of a protein or high-fibre snack (such as some chicken, a handful of almonds, or an apple) before you head out. Chapter 10 is all about surviving restaurants, special events and holidays.

✔ **Get regular exercise.** Exercise is as important to achieving optimal health as your nutrition and sleep. Regular exercise helps stave off sugar cravings, boosts your energy and tones your muscles. Exercise is essential for type 2 diabetics because it improves insulin sensitivity. Investigate Chapter 12 for an overview of constructing a basic exercise program that works for you.

✔ **Learn to identify and manage triggers and cravings.** If you're like most sugar addicts, you've learned to reach for something sweet under certain circumstances, like when you feel stressed, lonely, hungry or tired. To successfully reduce your sugar intake, you need to recognise these external triggers and practise making more conscious (and sensible) decisions when they present themselves. Chapter 9 — the most important chapter in this book, in our opinion — helps you determine what you really want when a craving hits.

✔ **Don't give up when you're not perfect.** People often get discouraged when they have a bad eating day, week or month. Keep this in mind: You can't fail at good nutrition because your nutrition can be simply rectified by awareness at your next meal. All you have to work with is what you choose to do *right now*, so don't beat yourself up because you've been less than perfect in the past. Check out Chapter 8 for an introduction to mindfulness and avoiding reactive behaviour.

Eating Right and Creating a New Normal

The reason diets don't work is that they don't lay out a realistic, sustainable plan that you can use to replace how you've been feeding yourself. Eating right doesn't require completely eliminating any one type of food (even sugar!) or some 'revolutionary' new system of nutrition. Your new normal should be about nourishing yourself with delicious, low-sugar foods — so much so that you forget about the unhealthy, ageing, health-sabotaging foods from your past.

Eating well, regaining mental and emotional clarity, and losing weight requires a series of small, ongoing decisions that replace what you used to do most of the time. Aristotle said that we are what we repeatedly do, so excellence is not a trait but a habit.

When you change what you usually do — that is, what's normal for you (see Chapter 9) — you get different results. No temporary diet can create a new normal for you; you must create one yourself by making different decisions most of the time.

Simplifying the low-carb concept

Perhaps you're a visual person, and images can often help to simplify a concept. So visualise yourself in a camp during the middle of winter. The night is freezing and you're going to sleep by the camp fire until morning. You can choose between two fires: One is a large fire made from lots of twigs and small bits of wood; the second fire is of equal size yet made from large logs, hearty timber. Which fire are you going to sleep by?

Of course, you'd choose the fire made from the hearty logs. They're long burners, so they provide sustaining energy and warmth. The twigs, however, are fast burners, so they provide only a quick release of energy and warmth, and then they're burnt out.

Complex carbohydrates (logs) assist in controlling your insulin levels. *Insulin* is a hormone that causes your cells to take up the glucose (sugar) that goes into the blood when you digest carbohydrates. Eating too many carbohydrates (or the wrong kind of carbohydrates — twigs) forces your body to produce a lot of insulin. Chronically high insulin levels cause conditions like metabolic syndrome, insulin resistance, type 2 diabetes, high cholesterol, PCOS and Alzheimer's disease. High insulin levels also promote fat storage and limit fat burning for energy. The primary way to keep your insulin levels low is to control your carbohydrate intake, both the type you choose (logs versus twigs) and the amount you eat. Look over Chapter 3 for an in-depth discussion on types of carbohydrates and insulin control.

All carbohydrates are broken down in your digestive system into simple sugars, but that doesn't mean that all carbohydrates are bad. If you're an active, thinking person, complex carbs can be used as fuel for your brain and muscles. Simple carbohydrates (twigs) break down faster and raise your blood sugar levels more than complex carbs (logs), which break down and release slowly. When it comes to blood sugar, slower is better. High blood sugar levels trigger a large insulin release, which causes fat storage, mood swings, tiredness and concentration problems, and, over time, can cause diabetes and serious tissue damage.

High-fibre carbohydrates (like vegetables, beans and complex grains) generally don't raise your blood sugar levels like sugary foods with no fibre (like lollies, soft drinks, white-flour foods, cakes, pies, biscuits and processed foods). Another way of keeping your blood sugar from spiking is to add quality proteins and fat into your meals. This addition of protein and fat drastically slows the rise of blood sugar from the carbs in that meal.

Improving your eating with five easy habits

Chapter 5 is all about putting together a healthy nutrition system for yourself. Here are some tips to get you started:

✔ Eating a high-protein breakfast stimulates your metabolism, stabilises your blood sugar and keeps your energy levels high throughout the morning. An all-carb continental breakfast promotes fat storage and puts you on the blood sugar roller-coaster for the rest of the day. See Chapter 13 for energy-boosting breakfast ideas.

✔ Vegetables should make up the majority of your carbohydrate intake (see Chapter 5). Vegetables are low in kilojoules and high in vitamins, minerals, fibre and phytonutrients, so they make the ideal carbohydrate choice. Fruits are high in nutrients, but they also contain more sugar, so be judicious in your portions.

✔ Try to eat a protein source every time you eat. Protein is essential for rebuilding muscles and organs and for making immune system cells, hormones, enzymes and a host of other necessary components of a healthy body. Eating protein with carbohydrates slows down the release of sugar into the bloodstream, so getting enough protein is important for blood sugar control too. Protein helps keep your appetite at bay longer than carbohydrates do.

✔ Drinking enough water is important to keep all your body's tissues healthy, including your brain. Being dehydrated decreases your mental and physical functions and triggers your hypothalamus to turn on the hunger and thirst centres in your brain, increasing appetite and cravings. A general guideline is to aim to drink a minimum of 1.5 litres of water every day.

✔ Using the right nutrition supplements is a good way to ensure that you supply your body with optimum nutrition. Nutrition deficiencies can cause food cravings and contribute to a host of degenerative diseases like arthritis, heart disease and cancer. Chapter 5 explains which nutrition supplements may be helpful under certain circumstances.

Change your thinking, change your life

Overcoming your sugar addiction requires different behaviours and new ways of thinking. You need to not only improve your nutrition plan but also train yourself to make proactive, conscious decisions instead of acting reactively to stress.

Learning to be mindful and intentional instead of being reactive is a crucial component of controlling your eating and managing the stress in your life. Your diet starts with your brain, not with your mouth, so go through Chapters 8 and 9 to begin changing your life by changing your thinking.

Figuring Out What You Really Need Instead of Sugar

If you're like most addicts, you use sugar to medicate yourself. Sugar is a substitute for something that's missing in your life. To stop the cravings and heal your addiction, you have to figure out what emotional 'hole' you're trying to fill with sugar.

The next time you have a craving for something sweet, stop to figure out what it is that you really want — chances are it's not sugar. Here are some examples:

✔ If you have the urge to grab something sweet when you get stressed, what you probably want is to feel peaceful and in control of your life. Sugar can't give you that.

✔ If you're ravenous when you get home at night and are ready to grab whatever you can stuff yourself with the fastest, what your body really wants is nourishment from real food. Sugar can't give you that.

✔ When you're ready to break into a vending machine full of chocolates and lollies because you had less than seven to eight hours of sleep, what you really need to figure out is why you're not sleeping enough. Sugar can't give you that.

✔ When you desire sugar because you feel lonely, sad or hopeless, what you probably want is companionship, hope and joy. Sugar can't give you that.

After you start to recognise what your real motivations are, you can start taking steps to achieve those states instead of drugging yourself with sugar. Chapter 9 takes you through the process in more detail.

Chapter 2

Figuring Out Why You're Addicted to Sugar

In This Chapter

▶ Understanding why sugar is so addictive

▶ Investigating different kinds of addicts

*I*n addition to being the driving force behind a multitude of health problems, sugar is a powerful, mood-altering substance that's as addictive as cocaine (more on that later in this chapter). No other food component affects your brain as strongly as sugar, and many people literally become addicted to the effects it has on brain chemistry.

Humans are prone to sugar addiction for many reasons. Everyone has a genetic predisposition to seek out the sweet stuff, and sugar (especially the processed kind) exerts strong effects on the brain and body chemistry that keep people hooked. Many people learn unhealthy eating cues and habits from their parents, and modern society makes sugar plentiful, cheap and enticing. Our goal for this book is to help you gain control over your eating, your health and your life!

In this chapter, we explore why sugar is so addictive and give you a glimpse into the behaviour and psychology of four typical types of sugar addict. You can take a quiz for each type of sugar addict to see how closely you resemble the common profile, and then follow the advice we give for each kind.

Getting to the Root of Why Sugar Is So Darned Addictive

Sugar addiction is prevalent in modern society because sugar is legal, cheap, pervasive and socially acceptable. You can't say that about the other substances people get addicted to. Combine all that with a stressful job, a busy family life and a full schedule, and is it any wonder that people stuff themselves with sugar-packed convenience foods?

But sugar's addictiveness isn't just a matter of social acceptance and availability. Sugar is physically addictive, affecting both the body and the brain. In this section, we cover some of the physical, emotional and social reasons sugar is so addictive.

Brain chemistry

Sugar (along with its addiction-prone cousins, starch, salt and fat) is one of the stimulating foodstuffs termed *hyperpalatables* — foods that stimulate the pleasure centres in the brain. Central to the brain's sensation of enjoyment is a chemical called *dopamine*, a neurotransmitter that controls the brain's reward and pleasure centres. When you eat sugar, it stimulates a dopamine release, and you experience a pleasurable sensation. It's easy for humans to get hooked on dopamine and consequently become addicted to the things that produce it — such as sugar, alcohol, cocaine, sex and methamphetamines.

Science shows that sugar acts on your brain's reward system just like cocaine. As with any dopamine-producing substance, your brain gets desensitised to it with chronic overconsumption, and you develop a tolerance. Therefore, if you want to create the pleasurable feeling, you have to use more and more. This launches a vicious cycle of increased consumption leading to further desensitisation, and you end up with an insatiable appetite for sugar (or whatever other substance you're abusing). At one time in your life, for example, two chocolate biscuits and a cup of tea may have dampened your sugar craving, but over time two may have turned into six!

Making matters more difficult, science has shown that as dopamine receptors decrease, a marked decrease also occurs in the activity of the *prefrontal cortex* — the part of your brain responsible for 'executive' functions like planning, organising and making rational decisions. This is a double-whammy for the sugar addict; not only do you have to eat more sugar to experience the normal reward and pleasure, but your addiction also makes it more difficult for your brain to plan ahead and make sensible food decisions!

Losing a sense of reasoning

Dopamine does more than just kick out pleasure signals. This neurotransmitter affects brain processes that control voluntary movement, emotional responses, motivation and the ability to anticipate rewards. Dopamine deficiency results in Parkinson's disease and has also been implicated in schizophrenia, ADHD and restless legs syndrome. Studies show that people with low dopamine activity appear to be more prone to addiction, and the presence of a certain kind of dopamine receptor is associated with sensation-seeking (addict) or thrill-seeking (adrenaline junkie) behaviour.

The feelings of satisfaction that dopamine exerts are so strong that, to obtain that satisfaction, an addict often loses the ability to reason. Because the brain develops neural circuits that unconsciously assess reward, addicts will do what they think is in their best interest, when in fact the only interest such behaviour satisfies is the release of dopamine. The unconscious need for the release of dopamine becomes all-important to the addict, and consequences and reason fly out the window.

Exercise not only improves the functioning of the prefrontal cortex but also directly regenerates dopamine receptors, helping to both rebuild the damage of past addiction and prevent it in the future! See Chapter 12 for some exercise tips.

Some nutritionists and health advocates are not surprised that governments are considering regulations on the amount of sugar in soft drinks and food items. After all, aren't cocaine, crack and methamphetamines illegal for adults — let alone children?

Genetic programming

Humans are programmed to utilise high-energy foods. Back in the cave-dwelling days, high-calorie foods meant a high chance of survival, so you're genetically programmed to prefer high-calorie foods (fat and sugar) over all others.

Over the last few years, some fascinating research has come to light in the field of *epigenetics* — the study of the body's chemistry that switches genes off and on. Not surprisingly, your diet and your environment change your body chemistry, and scientists are learning how this affects the switching on and off of certain genes that affect how your body processes food.

Here's a great example of a lifestyle that changes your gene expression to your detriment: You wake up already tired, hit the snooze button a few times, skip breakfast, and fly out the door after snapping at your kids and feeling awful about how fat you look in your outfit. Then you spend most of your day sitting glued to a computer screen in a stressed-out, fight-or-flight overdrive, trying to meet some deadline given to you by someone who doesn't understand you and doesn't care that you're surrounded by people who are just making your job harder. To anaesthetise the pain of this stressed-out existence and to quiet the part of your brain that's screaming for fuel, you grab whatever junk food is easily obtained nearby. This constant dependence on the quick sugar fix not only thickens your waistline but also changes your gene expression to one that supports fat storage and addiction. As Aristotle said, 'We are what we repeatedly do.'

Your DNA is not your destiny! You can't alter the genes you were born with, but you *can* change which of those genes express themselves by modifying how you eat and how you live. As you start to eat better and lead a healthier lifestyle, your gene expression will change to reflect the improvements in your body chemistry. Don't let your genes dictate your jeans!

Hunger and cravings

Leptin is a hormone that signals to your brain that you've had enough to eat, producing a sensation of fullness (satiety). Leptin is produced in the fat cells, so the more fat you have, the more leptin you produce. This is nature's way of keeping your weight under control. If you eat a normal, healthy diet, this system works fine, but unhealthy eating and lack of sleep can easily screw up the natural leptin-signalling system.

Nature's 'full' signal can get disrupted by many things, such as carrying too much body fat, maintaining chronically high insulin levels, ingesting too many artificial sweeteners, consuming excess sugar (especially fructose) or having elevated *triglycerides* (fat in your blood). When your leptin signals fail (a condition called *leptin resistance*), your hunger hormones run rampant and unopposed. This is why a consistent sugar overload, even though it provides you with calories and raises your blood sugar levels, stimulates hunger and cravings.

To reverse the hunger hormone tailspin that a high-sugar diet creates, you need to eat foods that promote satiety — quality proteins, good fats, fibrous vegetables, nuts and seeds (think of these as logs in your diet; refer to Chapter 1 for more). And you need to avoid foods that raise insulin — sugar, fructose, sweetened drinks and processed grains (think of these as twigs). Exercise, weight loss and sleep both boost the effectiveness and sensitivity of insulin and leptin.

Feeding yeast infections

A yeast infection is an overgrowth of one or more of the naturally occurring fungi (typically the *Candida albicans* yeast) that inhabit dark, moist parts of your body. Your immune system usually keeps *Candida* from growing out of control, but if the immune system is compromised, an overgrowth can occur.

A high-sugar diet lowers your immune system's power (see Chapter 4 for more on the immune system) and reduces the amount of beneficial bacteria in your intestines (which further weakens the immune system). Yeast feeds on sugar, and yeast grows best in an acidic environment. Eating lots of sugar gives the yeast both of those conditions.

Because yeast feeds on sugar, it typically triggers very strong cravings for sugar (and sometimes alcohol). This starts a vicious cycle; the more sugar you eat, the more yeast grows, and the stronger the cravings become. (Perhaps you're nodding your head as you read this, because you've experienced exactly this type of vicious cravings cycle.)

Antibiotic use kills off bad bacteria but unfortunately also kills the beneficial bacteria in your intestines (the *intestinal flora*), giving yeast and other opportunistic microorganisms a big 'Vacancy' sign. After a course of antibiotics, it's important to replace the beneficial bacteria with a good probiotic supplement (see Chapter 5 for the scoop on probiotics).

Recurring yeast infections are a red flag that your body is not in balance, which could have long-term consequences. If left untreated, frequent or persistent yeast infections can damage the intestines, overtax the immune system, cause systemic inflammation, and spread to other organs and tissues. They are also often a warning of high glucose levels, which may be leading to type 2 diabetes. If you're prone to yeast infections, you need to change to a low-sugar diet immediately and to begin a course of probiotic therapy that's right for your personal health history. Consult a knowledgeable healthcare practitioner for guidance and a holistic approach — if he gives you an antibiotic or antifungal medication and sends you on your way without any discussion of diet and probiotics, seek out a more knowledgeable practitioner (see Chapter 7 for some healthcare practitioner advice).

Learned behaviour

Humans are creatures of habit. Food preferences start early in life and, after children develop the habit of eating sugar, fat and salt, they get locked into a self-perpetuating cycle of preferring these foods into adulthood (scientists call this *pervasive palate preference*). Your love affair with sugar probably started at an early age and was perpetuated by your parents' eating habits. As a child, your parents or grandparents may have given you sweets as a reward or as a distraction to calm you down. As an adult, this naturally becomes an emotional crutch if you still equate sugar with being good or being calm.

Associating certain events with sugar is another thing that most people learn over their lifetime. Cake is typically a centrepiece of birthdays, weddings, retirement parties and the like. Holiday celebrations such as Easter, Christmas and New Year's Day often include lots of sweets. (Some people think not having a pavlova on Australia Day or an Anzac biscuit on Anzac day is 'unAustralian'. Or that not eating hokey-pokey ice-cream should get you deported from New Zealand.) See Chapter 10 for tips on surviving holidays and special occasions.

Many addicts learn to reach for sugar as an attempt to avoid negative feelings like stress, loneliness or low self-esteem. These habits quickly become destructive, addictive behaviours as you learn to use a sugar coma to squelch genuine emotions that desperately need your attention.

Polite conventions in society tend to perpetuate sugar abuse. If you have people to your house for dinner, you naturally assume you have to serve them dessert, right? And as the guest, you feel obligated to eat it even if you don't want it because you don't want to appear rude. Offering an addictive drug to your guests would be bizarre, but offering (and accepting) sugar appears to be obligatory.

By using the techniques in this book to change how you view sugar and how you plan your food, you can unlearn the unhealthy programming, remain aware of your triggers, and stay in control of your own behaviour.

What Kind of Sugarholic Are You?

The following sections outline the four main types of sugar addict and explain some general behaviour and psychology traits common to each one. If you understand what kind of sugar addict you are and you learn to recognise some behaviours and thought patterns common to each addict type, you may start to understand how you've become addicted to sugar. Even more important, you'll discover what you need to do to overcome your addiction and regain control of your life.

Answer the questions for each quiz using the following scoring system:

> 0 points for 'Never'
>
> 2 points for 'Sometimes, but rarely'
>
> 5 points for 'Half the time'
>
> 10 points for 'Most of the time' or 'Always'

If you'd like more information to help you evaluate whether you're addicted to sugar, turn to Chapter 1.

The Exhausted Addict

To determine how closely you resemble the classic Exhausted Addict, take the following quiz using the scoring system at the beginning of this section.

_____ Do you need caffeine to get started in the morning and/or to make it through the day?

_____ Do you have trouble going to sleep, or do you wake up in the middle of the night without being able to go back to sleep?

_____ Do you eat your sugar fix so quickly you don't even remember enjoying the flavours?

_____ Do you crave sweets when you get tired?

_____ Do you experience indigestion or acid reflux?

_____ Do you feel like you're always running — that you never have enough hours in the day?

_____ Do you have chronic aches, pains and tight muscles?

_____ Do you get headaches?

_____ Do you put others' needs above your own?

_____ Do you think that if you don't do it, it won't get done?

_____ Do you eat sugar or fast food because you don't have time for something healthy?

Now add up your score:

0–30 points: You don't show strong signs of being an Exhausted Addict.

31–50 points: You exhibit some of the Exhausted Addict symptoms. Chances are you'll score similarly for at least one other type of addict.

51–100 points: You fit the mould of the classic Exhausted Addict. Read on and see whether the following description of the typical Exhausted Addict's personality sounds like you.

Understanding the Exhausted Addict

If you're an Exhausted Addict, you're the epitome of someone who runs too hard. You don't know the meaning of the word _downtime_, and fatigue is almost constant. You never seem to have enough hours in the day to get everything done, and you pressure yourself to try to be the one who does everything for everyone except yourself.

Exhausted Addicts are generally perfectionists who can't accept anything except the best from themselves. You see yourself as the go-to person when a crisis arises, and you create an unhealthy sense of pride by ignoring your own self-care and putting everyone else's needs before your own.

Exhausted Addicts regularly have sore muscles, trigger points and areas that stay tight and painful. Stress and poor breathing habits keep muscles tight and turned on when they shouldn't be. Painful knots and trigger points develop, and, with an overactive nervous system, this can progress to chronic muscular issues (see Chapter 4). Exhausted Addicts don't recognise that these muscle aches and pains, and the general feeling of exhaustion are leading to bigger disease processes — often until it's too late.

Due to stresses (both external and self-created), marginal diet and lack of sleep, the Exhausted Addict's adrenal function becomes impaired (see Chapter 4). This is referred to as *adrenal fatigue*, and it results in chronic fatigue, low thyroid function and low blood sugar that triggers sugar cravings.

Exhausted Addicts tend to eat poorly because they think planning their eating requires too much time and attention. Instead of sitting down for a healthy meal, these types of addict grab whatever's handy, often turning to sugar or other junk food to give them the energy boost they desperately need.

The stress from the Exhausted Addict's punishing schedule causes insomnia and restless sleep. Lack of sleep disrupts the normal production of appetite-suppressing hormones, so the Exhausted Addict is prone to hunger and cravings. If you reach for the sugar when this happens, you'll find that, like most other addicts of this type, your waist has expanded even though you may not have gained weight in other parts of your body.

Advice for the Exhausted Addict

In addition to weaning themselves off sugar with the techniques in Part III, Exhausted Addicts can benefit from learning to *plan* instead of *react*. Because the Exhausted Addict's life feels so out of control and pressured, any amount of pre-planned control helps reduce stress levels and improve eating habits. Ask yourself: Have you achieved recognition for anything that you're proud of that hasn't required planning? See Chapter 8 for tips on planning and eating mindfully instead of reactively.

The Sad Eater

To determine how closely you resemble the classic Sad Eater, take the following quiz using the scoring system at the beginning of this section.

_____ Are you lonely?

_____ Do you find yourself wishing your life were drastically different?

_____ Do you have a decreased sex drive?

_____ Do you tend to do the same things week in and week out?

_____ Do you have strong PMS symptoms?

_____ Do you turn to sugar or other comfort foods when you feel sad or lonely?

_____ Do you wake up tired no matter how long you've slept?

_____ Do you watch more than one hour of television per night?

_____ Do you feel depressed or hopeless and hardly exercise?

_____ Do you eat sugar late at night, regardless of whether you're hungry or not?

Now tally up your score:

> 0–25 points: You don't show strong signs of being a Sad Eater.
>
> 26–50 points: You exhibit some of the Sad Eater symptoms. Chances are you'll score similarly for at least one other type of addict.
>
> 51–100 points: You fit the mould of the classic Sad Eater. Read on and see whether the following description of the typical Sad Eater's personality sounds like you.

Understanding the Sad Eater

As the name implies, Sad Eaters spend a lot of time feeling sad and depressed. They use sugar as an artificial mood elevator, and their behaviours with food embody the very definition of the term *emotional eater*. Out of all the addict types, the Sad Eater has the unhealthiest relationship with food. It's common for Sad Eaters to turn to sugar for comfort and companionship; often, Sad Eaters feel like food is their only friend, even if they're surrounded by family or co-workers.

Sad Eaters often have a strong *inner critic* (see Chapter 9), and can have self-esteem issues. Many Sad Eaters find themselves in a difficult catch-22 with food — they feel unhealthy, overweight and unlovable, so they eat sugar for comfort, telling themselves they 'just don't care'. And for that moment that they are eating, they *don't* care. But then they sink further into the Sad Eater mentality and self-dislike after their binge — a self-sabotaging cycle.

Sad Eaters are often angry, crabby and/or judgemental toward others. If you find yourself regularly getting irritated with co-workers or angry with family members because they don't act according to your expectations, you may be exhibiting Sad Eater behaviour.

Sad Eaters may be peri-menopausal or are particularly sensitive to PMS and monthly hormone fluctuations. Sugar depletes many nutrients and can unbalance neurotransmitters as well as sex hormones. Hormone deficiencies and imbalances can wreak havoc with Sad Eaters' emotional state. If you have a deficiency of oestrogen, progesterone and/or testosterone, you can become sad or even clinically depressed. When this happens, you start to crave sugar in an attempt to raise your serotonin levels (see Chapter 4 for more on serotonin).

Advice for the Sad Eater

Sad Eaters can more easily stay away from sugar if they develop a better sense of emotional awareness. Become aware: Aware of your triggers, aware of what you're putting in your mouth, aware of your self-sabotage. Do some self-inquiry to uncover more details about the negative emotions that you're experiencing — the more specific the better. For example, if you're feeling stressed at work, try to find someone to whom you can describe what you're feeling. One of the big successes of Alcoholics Anonymous is that the reforming alcoholics have a mate who they can call on when they need it. Find someone who you can confide in and who will be encouraging of you making healthy changes. Instead of just telling your support person you're stressed out, explain the feeling. Do you feel overwhelmed? Unappreciated? Afraid? Trapped? Inadequate? When you start to understand a more detailed picture of your reactions and emotions, you're able to more accurately assess the situation and deal with the truth instead of just reacting negatively and reaching for the sweet drug.

Some professional therapy can help steer the Sad Eater toward greater emotional awareness. See Chapter 11 for tips on seeking out support groups and professional help.

In addition to weaning yourself off sugar with the tools in Part III, Sad Eaters need to put extra effort and attention on the substitute behaviours covered in Chapter 9. The best things to boost a Sad Eater's mood are to do something outside the normal routine and to do something good for someone else.

The Numb Eater

To determine how closely you resemble the classic Numb Eater, take the following quiz using the scoring system at the beginning of this section.

_____ Are you tired most of the day?

_____ When something stressful happens to you, does your energy nose-dive and you quickly feel like giving up?

_____ Do you skip breakfast?

_____ Do you eat a low-protein diet (only one or two protein servings per day)? See Chapter 5 if you're not sure what constitutes a serving of protein.

_____ Do you have cravings at night but are ambivalent about food during the day?

_____ Do you drink less than eight glasses of water per day?

_____ Do you eat inconsistently, eating a majority of your food for the day after 5 pm?

_____ Do you need caffeine to stay alert in the middle of the day?

_____ Do you have trouble concentrating, with brain fog overwhelming your thoughts more than once per day?

_____ Do you get irritable with people?

Now tally up your score:

> 0–25 points: You don't show signs of being a classic Numb Eater.

> 26–45 points: You exhibit some signs of being a Numb Eater. Chances are you'll score similarly for at least one other type of addict.

> 46–100 points: You definitely fit the mould of the classic Numb Eater. Read on and see whether the following description of the typical Numb Eater's personality sounds like yours.

Understanding the Numb Eater

The classic Numb Eater is often a low-energy person, numb to seeing enjoyment in life. You love to sleep, and you generally find it very difficult to muster the energy to do anything above and beyond what is absolutely necessary — even things you enjoy. In that respect, Numb Eaters are similar to Exhausted Addicts (discussed earlier in this section), but while Exhausted Addicts continue to unhealthily push themselves through their stress and exhaustion, Numb Eaters crash and shut down instead.

If you're a Numb Eater, you probably have a history of spinning your wheels and feeling stuck or trapped in your job, your family issues and your body size. Numb Eaters often feel out of touch with others and regularly ignore or feel numb about their own emotional problems, admitting that 'I just can't deal with that right now'.

You seldom eat breakfast and, when you do, it's usually an all-carb affair. In fact, most of your food is carbohydrate. You tell yourself that you eat enough protein 'on most days', but if you journal your food for a few days, you'll see that you barely eat one or two servings of protein a day — not even enough to meet the recommended daily intake, let alone enough to be healthy and energetic. Eating like this keeps your metabolism low, so you probably find yourself gaining weight even though you don't eat much.

Like many sugar addicts, the Numb Eater feels overwhelmed with making food choices. You've tried dozens of frustrating diets and special 'detoxes' over the years, none of which has yielded any long-term success. Eating healthily takes too much thinking and planning, so like the Exhausted Addict, you turn to processed, convenient, sugary foods because they're easy.

Advice for the Numb Eater

By beginning to wean yourself off sugar, you'll start to feel more energetic and feel like you have more control over your food choices. In addition to following the how-to advice in Part III of this book, the best advice we have for the Numb Eater is:

- Make sure you eat protein at every meal.

- When you have a sugar craving, get up and *do* something! Your body and your brain are craving activity and stimulation, so take a walk, do breathing exercises, write in your journal, take a bath, phone a friend, plan your weekend, search for a healthy recipe online — anything rather than continuing to drug yourself with sugar.

The Sugar Stalker

To determine how closely you resemble the classic Sugar Stalker, take the following quiz using the scoring system at the beginning of this section.

____ Do you keep a stash of sweets at work or in the pantry at home?

____ Do you drink sweetened drinks?

____ Do you get headaches or become irritable if you skip your sugar fix?

____ Do you eat sweet things like pastries or doughnuts first thing in the day?

___ When you start eating sugar, do you have trouble stopping?

___ Do you have a craving for something sweet after every meal?

___ Do you become stressed when you think about changing your eating habits?

___ Are you a chocoholic?

___ Do you hide sweets or are you embarrassed to eat them in front of others?

___ Do you order dessert at a restaurant even if you're full?

Now add up your score:

0–30 points: You don't show strong signs of being a Sugar Stalker.

31–50 points: You exhibit some of the Sugar Stalker symptoms. Chances are you'll score similarly for at least one other type of addict.

51–100 points: You behave like the classic Sugar Stalker. Read on and see whether the following description of the typical Sugar Stalker sounds like you.

Understanding the Sugar Stalker

Out of all the addicts, the Sugar Stalker is the most physically addicted to sugar — meaning true chemical/physiological addiction. The Sugar Stalker's taste buds have been overstimulated and desensitised to the point of finding nothing but the most over-sugared, sickly-sweet treats to be even remotely satisfying.

If you're a Sugar Stalker, your life revolves around sugar to the point where your eyes light up and your mouth starts to water at the very mention of something sweet. Sugar Stalkers eat a stream of sugar throughout the day, starting with a high-sugar breakfast of sweetened coffee, pastries or fruit juice. Sweet snacks like lollies and biscuits are the norm, and the thought of drinking something that isn't sweetened — even water — turns their stomach, even if they're thirsty.

Sugar Stalkers, like many people addicted to a given substance, act impulsively when presented with their object of addiction. They're always scheming up ways to eat more sugar without anyone noticing, taking a second handful of lollies and hoping no-one sees them, gulping down chocolates in the pantry or behind the refrigerator door. They often eat in their cars and hide the wrappers from others and themselves.

Interestingly, Sugar Stalkers may appear confident, but often are vulnerable and suffer from self-esteem problems.

Advice for the Sugar Stalker

If you're a Sugar Stalker, you need to give up sweetened drinks and artificial sweeteners as soon as possible. Your taste buds and the dopamine reward centre in your brain need to be re-sensitised to what normal food tastes like, and sweet drinks — even diet soft drinks with no actual sugar — make that impossible. When you feed your body an artificial sweetener that is hundreds of times sweeter than natural sugars, your tastes buds sense the sweet taste and activate insulin — your fat storage hormone (see Chapter 3 for more on this). This just perpetuates the vicious sugar addict cycle you are in.

See Chapter 9 for ideas about substitute beverages and for a step-by-step guide on what to do when a sugar craving strikes.

In addition to becoming a disciple of Chapter 9, you need to redefine dessert. To gradually disengage from the habit of having to have something sweet after every meal, start by substituting sweet things that are healthier — for example, a few berries, some plain yoghurt, or simply a naturally sweet herbal tea such as licorice, cinnamon or lemongrass. Michele's personal sweet treat is raw cocoa powder and some shredded coconut stirred into a bit of coconut oil — the dark bitter flavour of the cocoa mixed with the oily tasty fat of the coconut and coconut oil satisfies your sweet cravings yet provides lots of nutrients without any sugar!

Portion control is another thing that helps you get off sugar (see Chapter 5 for more on portion control). If you're a Sugar Stalker, it's important for you to create awareness about your portion size — even the size of your healthy meals and snacks. Getting rid of portion distortion means never eating from a package and putting your food on a plate instead — and walking away after your meal to remove additional temptation.

Try one piece (and only one!) of dark chocolate (70 per cent cocoa or more), and let it melt in your mouth. It may take a little bit of time to acquire a taste for dark chocolate, but probably not too long if you're missing milk chocolate!

Only allow yourself a taste of something sweet once you've successfully kicked sugar out. We find that most people need to be a bit strict with themselves through the transition period to a low-sugar way of life (the length of the transition period varies for everyone but is usually between two and four weeks). Once you feel in control of your sweet tooth, you may opt for some dark chocolate in small portions.

Chapter 3

The Lowdown on Sugar and Carbs

*Y*our body doesn't deal with all carbohydrates in the same fashion. Different types of carbs have different effects on your body chemistry. Overcoming your sugar addiction requires the ability to evaluate carbohydrates, and an understanding of how the choices you make affect your body and your brain.

Information about sugar and low-carb eating can be confusing, so this chapter delivers the simple facts on carbohydrates and sugars (without too much biochemistry), how your body processes them, and how you can distinguish good carbs from bad carbs.

One of the common approaches for attempting to reduce carbohydrate intake is to eliminate gluten from the diet. Though gluten doesn't have anything to do with sugar addiction, some people have an easier time cutting back on their total carb intake if they stop eating gluten-based foods such as wheat, rye and barley. In particular, some people find excluding bread helps with reducing carbs. So, we dedicate a section of this chapter to guiding you through the basic principles of going gluten-free.

To make a responsible nutrition plan, recognising where your sugar intake comes from is important. This chapter discusses some common sources of dietary sugar, including many hidden sources of which you may not be aware. Finally, we include important information for you and your loved ones — the shocking truth about the dangers of artificial sweeteners.

Sugar: The New Poison

The epidemic of obesity and diabetes in the Western world has three main causes: the sugar content in food, inactivity, and increased overall calorie consumption. Combining all three, as has happened over the years, creates the perfect storm for a health and wellness catastrophe. Additionally, as more people become overweight or obese, people — including children and their parents — become less aware of what a normal, healthy weight is. Overweight or obese becomes the norm.

Sugar abuse can lead to myriad health problems, including weight gain, diabetes, depressed immunity, elevated cholesterol and triglycerides, cancer, tooth decay, yeast infections, liver disease, depression, chronic fatigue, increased appetite and metabolic syndrome. If a pharmaceutical company put a pill on chemist shelves that could cause all those side effects, an outcry would ensue — followed by quick action to get the pill removed from the public's reach!

But sugar is a food product, even though it has drug-like effects. It's cheap, it's abundant and people *love it*. Sugar is pervasive in our society, and therein lies the problem.

The biggest culprits in the Western food supply are soft drinks, cordials, lollies, and commercially processed and baked goods. Those account for approximately three-quarters of the total sugar that people consume. So by cutting out junk food like that, you can easily reduce your sugar consumption by 75 per cent!

The Science of Carbohydrates

Carbohydrates — you hear and read the word all the time. Good carbs, bad carbs, low carb, high carb, sugary carbs, carb phobia — what does it all mean?

In a nutshell, a *carbohydrate* is any one of a group of compounds that includes sugars, starches and cellulose (fibre). Your body digests the carbohydrates that you eat and breaks them down into a sugar called *glucose*, which is the preferred form of carbohydrate that the body uses for fuel.

Identifying sources of carbohydrates

Many people mistakenly think of carbohydrates as only starches (pasta, bread, potatoes and so on) and sweets. But you find carbs in a variety of other foods. Here's a quick list of dietary sources of carbohydrates:

- ✔ Fruits
- ✔ Grain products like breads, cereals and pastas
- ✔ Sugars like lollies, honey, sweetened beverages, syrups and table sugar
- ✔ Vegetables

A good rule is if the carbohydrate is inside a box, bag and/or wrapper, it's often processed with hidden sugars.

Seeing why sugar is so bad for you

Carbohydrates are very important to living beings. You need carbohydrates in your diet to provide energy to each cell, to supply your brain with glucose, and to furnish fuel for your muscles and organs. All your DNA and RNA molecules have a sugar molecule (ribose) in them. In fact, if you don't eat enough carbohydrates, your body breaks down protein from muscle tissue to make some!

So if carbohydrates are so important, why is sugar so bad for you? What's with all the low-carb buzz?

The physiological response you get from eating any carbohydrate depends on the *type* of carb and the *amount* that you eat. Do it right and you have a normal, healthy response. Do it wrong and the chemistry created in your body makes you fat, sick and addicted.

Your body uses the energy it gets from carbohydrates to do various important jobs — feed the brain, make cells do their thing, and fill up your muscles and organs with fuel. After these jobs are finished, your body promptly packages up and stores any leftover carbs as body fat.

Note: From here in this book, we use the word *sugar* to mean a food that is a low-nutrient, fibre-free carbohydrate like lollies, high-fructose corn syrup, sweetened soft drinks and table sugar, even though other types of carbohydrates are technically broken down into sugars too.

The problem with sugar is that it's not only high in calories but also virtually nutrient- and fibre-free. When you eat a lot of sugar (especially without fibre, protein or fat), far too much sugar enters the bloodstream at one time. This creates a blood sugar high in your body, which responds to the assault by prompting the pancreas to release a large dose of insulin to attempt to control the sugar levels. When our blood sugar roller-coasters to a high, it will equally come roller-coastering down causing mood swings, severe hunger, sweats, exhaustion and more.

Connecting carbs and sugar to insulin

Type 2 diabetes is one of the biggest threats to modern human health. With high sugar intake, low amounts of exercise and too many calories overall (which unfortunately describes many Australians and New Zealanders these days), the body is forced to produce more and more *insulin*, a hormone that's essential for preventing a dangerous build-up of sugar in your bloodstream but that, at high levels, can cause problems.

High insulin levels cause you to store fat and crave more food. This cycle continues over the years and, as you gain weight, your body becomes less and less sensitive to insulin, and it craves more and more sugar. The end result is obesity and insulin resistance, which lead to type 2 diabetes. (Chapter 4 tells you more about diabetes and other health problems linked to sugar.)

The most important source of fuel for your body is glucose, which enters the bloodstream after you eat. Glucose then travels throughout your bloodstream and is used by every cell in your body for energy, including your brain.

The pancreas, an organ located behind your stomach, is in charge of releasing hormones that make your body either store or release kilojoules. One of those hormones is insulin.

Insulin 'unlocks' your cells to allow the glucose circulating in the blood to enter the cells, where it can be turned into energy. After you eat a meal, your pancreas senses a rise in your blood sugar level and releases the insulin needed to move sugar from your blood into your cells. When you eat too many carbohydrates (especially sugars and low-fibre carbs), your pancreas is forced to secrete a lot of insulin to manage all that sugar.

Insulin generally does an adequate job of shuttling sugar to the right places (including turning all the extra sugar into fat), but regularly having high insulin levels may cause several serious problems:

- High insulin levels decrease your ability to burn body fat for fuel.

- Over time, your body becomes less sensitive to all the extra insulin, and so the insulin stops doing its job of letting in the glucose (the fuel for cells). This is called *insulin resistance*, and the fuel not getting into your cells makes you sleepy and sluggish. Not only are your cells not getting the required glucose, but they're also not getting the nutrients that accompany the glucose. You're starving and your cells are too — literally!

✔ High insulin levels lower blood sugar levels — that's insulin's job if it's working effectively. However, too much insulin lowers blood sugar levels too far and a sugar crash (*hypoglycaemic situation*) can occur. This can cause more cravings, severe brain fog, greater mood swings and mindless eating, which restarts the sugar roller-coaster cycle all over again.

✔ Insulin resistance inevitably leads to type 2 diabetes and/or metabolic syndrome.

Carbs versus Undesirable Carbs

Not all carbohydrates are the same and, despite what some mainstream diets pronounce, not every carbohydrate is your enemy. Now that you understand how insulin works (refer to the preceding section), it's time to discover how to select carbohydrates that give you a slow release of glucose into the body.

Separating complex carbs from simple carbs

As a general rule, the more stuff the digestive system has to break down, the more gradual the sugar release into the bloodstream is. Slower is better because a slower sugar release means you produce less insulin. For a healthy insulin response, you should choose carbohydrates that are *complex* — carbs that are made up of long chains of sugar molecules and that, therefore, take longer to break down. Compare the sustaining power, energy, heat and usefulness of a hearty log (complex carb) with a fast burning, unsustaining twig (simple carb) — refer to Chapter 1 for more on this log versus twig analogy. Examples of complex carbohydrates are fibrous vegetables like sweet potatoes, broccoli and green beans and wholegrain starches like brown rice, buckwheat, quinoa and whole-wheat.

 To further slow down sugar release, try to eat protein and fat with those complex carbohydrates! This is a particularly good strategy for those who always feel hungry.

Simple carbohydrates consist of only one or two molecules and thus break down and enter the bloodstream very quickly. This makes the pancreas release a lot of insulin to control the rapid rise in sugar levels. High insulin levels cause many problems, so try to stay away from simple carbs. Simple carbohydrates are sugars, most commercially processed bakery goods, and sweet stuff like lollies, corn syrup, fruit juice, soft drinks, cordials and sports drinks.

Getting more fibre and nutrition per kilojoule

The best kinds of carbohydrates are the ones that contain fibre, are low in sugar, and are nutrient-dense.

So, generally, vegetables are perfect. A good rule to keep in mind is that the darker a vegetable or grain is, the more nutrients it contains. Dark, leafy greens are more nutritious than white iceberg lettuce. Quinoa, brown rice and wild rice have more nutrients than white rice.

Most of your carbohydrates should come from vegetables because they're high in fibre and nutrients, yet low in sugar — you can eat a large volume of vegetables without consuming too many total carbohydrates. Be conscious that sweet corn and white potatoes are higher in carbs than other vegetables, so don't be excessive with them.

To generalise, you can pretty much eat all the vegetables you want without getting into too much trouble — we have never met an obese person who only eats vegetables.

If you have gastrointestinal issues like Crohn's disease or irritable bowel syndrome (IBS), you may need to temper the amount of fibre you consume. Readers with these medical conditions should consult a qualified professional for personalised advice.

Fruits are high in vitamins and minerals, but they're also higher in kilojoules and sugar (fructose) than vegetables, so be judicious in your consumption. Avoid drinking fruit juice because it's basically fibre-free and very high in sugar. Enjoy one entire piece of fruit instead of the five (or perhaps more) pieces that have been juiced, stripped of fibre and put in a plastic bottle.

Addressing problems with fructose

As we mention earlier in the chapter, not all carbohydrates are the same. A particular kind of sugar called *fructose* is particularly troublesome in the Western diet.

Excess sugar of any form — whether from fructose or glucose — is not beneficial to your health. If you want to break your sugar addiction, keep in mind that any sweet will trigger sweet cravings, regardless of whether that sweet is from fructose, glucose or an artificial sweetener.

Fructose occurs naturally in fruit. From that source it generally isn't a problem because, in natural foods and combined with fibre, fructose is not as problematic for the liver. The fructose that you find in manufactured foods, however, perpetuates sugar binging and doesn't do you any good at all.

Fructose being used as a prevalent sweetener (agave nectar, crystalline fructose, high-fructose corn syrup, honey and so on) is what makes it a biological problem. Humans can digest only a small amount of fructose, but many Australians and New Zealanders are binging on up to 75 grams of fructose per day, without really being aware they are doing so. Eating too much fructose can cause bloating, flatulence, loose stools and, on a deeper level, liver dysfunction.

Overconsumption of fructose is also a major factor in weight gain. The process of digestion breaks down most carbohydrates into glucose, which is the most basic fuel on the planet. All your cells use it, so your body processes it efficiently because it goes literally everywhere in the body. Fructose, however, is a very different simple sugar that isn't used in cells in the same way as other sugars. All fructose goes to the liver, where most of it is immediately converted into triglycerides (fat). When you consistently eat a lot of fructose, you not only overload your liver (causing non-alcoholic fatty liver disease) but also basically create body fat.

Here are some more problems with consuming large amounts of fructose:

- ✔ **Cardiovascular problems:** Excess fructose in the diet causes elevated cholesterol, homocysteine and triglyceride levels.

- ✔ **Leptin insensitivity:** Fructose doesn't stimulate the production of *leptin*, an appetite-suppressing hormone, like other carbohydrates do. The brain, unable to recognise that leptin is present, responds as if the body is starving. It then signals the body to lower the rate of metabolism and to store any fat that happens to be in the food. Hence, a high-fructose diet leads to extra storage of dietary fat and increased appetite.

- ✔ **Toxic by-products:** The liver's metabolism of fructose creates a long list of waste products and toxins, including a large amount of uric acid, which increases blood pressure and can cause gout and other arthritic symptoms.

Food manufacturers in Australia and New Zealand don't use the enormous amount of high-fructose corn syrup that American manufacturers do. However, according to the *American Journal of Clinical Nutrition*, corn syrup sweeteners now represent more than 20 per cent of the total daily carbohydrate intake for an average American. With Australians' and Kiwis' love of imported confectionery and sweet biscuits, this doesn't leave us far behind. Become a label reader!

Current research shows that approximately half of the population is unable to digest 25 grams of fructose by itself. Naturally occurring fructose (found in fruit) is bound with glucose, making absorption a non-issue in reasonable amounts. For example, a couple of pieces of fruit per day equals about 10 grams of fructose and will not cause long-term liver damage. Processed fructose (like high-fructose corn syrup and crystalline fructose) is a different story. You often find high levels of fructose in soft drinks, cordials, fruit juice, canned fruit, fruit jam, commercial bakery goods, sauces and condiments, and sweetened cereals. This type of sugar can easily overload the liver. You should limit your consumption of fructose (especially the artificial kind!), and if you have to eat it, don't exceed 25 grams unless you're prepared for long-term damage.

What about alcohol?

Alcoholic drinks generally contain only small amounts of sugar (assuming that you don't add lots of a sugary mixer). Even a glass of sweet white wine usually contains only about 8 grams of sugar. But be careful — this doesn't mean that the wine is low in kilojoules. Most alcoholic beverages consist of mostly high-glycaemic carbohydrates.

Despite its relatively low sugar content, alcohol can have a drastic effect on your blood sugar levels. Although alcohol may cause a slight rise in blood sugar levels when you initially ingest it, the overall effect of alcohol is to cause a drop in blood sugar. Normally, when your blood sugar starts to drop, your liver starts utilising its stored carbs, turning them into glucose for energy. However, when alcohol enters the system, your body reacts like the alcohol is a toxin that it wants to clear quickly from the blood. The liver is busy getting rid of the alcohol and so won't produce more glucose (from the stored carbs) until the alcohol is cleared; hence, blood glucose falls. This is why it's important not to drink on an empty stomach.

The more you drink, the more your blood sugar drops. Drinking as little as 60 millilitres of alcohol on an empty stomach can lead to a very low blood sugar level, which can be a big problem for anyone with diabetes. It also increases your appetite and lowers your will-power, as anyone who has had too much to drink can attest to.

Over time, excessive alcohol consumption can decrease insulin's effectiveness, resulting in high blood sugar levels and insulin resistance. One study showed that 70 per cent of people with alcoholic liver disease had either glucose intolerance or diabetes.

Food manufacturers have recently begun using sugar alcohols as sweeteners. *Sugar alcohols* are technically neither sugars nor alcohols; they're carbohydrates with a chemical structure that partially resembles sugar and partially resembles alcohol (but they don't contain ethanol, like alcoholic beverages do). *Polyols*, as sugar alcohols are also known, aren't completely absorbed and metabolised by the body and consequently contribute about 25 per cent fewer calories than most sugars — but you should still consider them sugar. Many sugar alcohols have unpleasant side effects, including flatulence, bloating, stomach cramps and diarrhoea. Commonly used sugar alcohols include erythritol, isomalt, lactitol, maltitol, maltitol syrup, mannitol, sorbitol and xylitol — these are best avoided.

Making substitutions for better carbs and less sugar

One of the easiest things you can do to reduce your sugar intake and keep your insulin levels under control is to substitute healthier carbohydrates for the ones containing more sugar and less fibre.

Table 3-1 can help you make some smart substitutions in your day-to-day food decisions.

Table 3-1	Substituting Smarter Carbs for Sugary Carbs
Instead of This	**Eat This**
White pasta	Brown rice pasta Whole-wheat pasta Wild rice Quinoa
Fruit juice or cordial	Teas such as green tea, lemongrass tea, licorice tea, rooibos tea Sparkling water with lemon
Cappuccino or Latte with sugar	Espresso or coffee without sweetener or with stevia*
Jams, conserves or marmalades	Strawberry slices Blueberries Vegemite Nut butters such as peanut butter or almond butter, without added sugar
Corn flakes and commercial cereals	Slow-cooked or traditional (not instant) oats or muesli without dried fruit
Soft drink	Mineral water with citrus slices
Sweets	Dark chocolate (minimum 70% cocoa)
After-dinner treat	Plain yoghurt with berries or a seed mixture on top
White bread	Wholegrain bread, rye, pumpernickel, buckwheat, amaranth (and half the amount)
White rice	Quinoa Brown rice Basmati rice
Mid-afternoon junk food	Crunchy raw vegetables with hummus or avocado dip Baked corn chips with salsa Smoothie with milk and frozen berries Piece of cheese

(continued)

Table 3-1   *(continued)*

Instead of This	Eat This
Takeaway breakfast muffin	Homemade muffin One slice of wholegrain toast topped with two poached or hard-boiled eggs
Commercial trail mix	Handful of almonds or walnuts (or any nuts that are raw — not roasted, oiled and salted)
Meat pie	Seeded crackers or wholegrain bread roll with cheese
Puddings	Cottage cheese, coconut milk pudding
Cake or dessert	Bowl of berries with cream on top A few pieces of cheese
Ice-cream	Non-GMO popcorn (popped yourself, not commercial microwave 'popcorn' in a bag)

Stevia is a plant-based sweetener that might help you through your transition to a low-sugar lifestyle.

Reading the labels on prepared or packaged foods is important — what may seem like a healthy choice may be the opposite. For example, many commercial nut, fruit and dried fruit mixes are loaded with dried fruit, which is high in sugar and chemicals. And bread with 'whole-wheat' on the package may not truly be whole-wheat — it might also contain plain white flour. Flip to Chapter 6 for more info about reading labels.

Understanding Where Your Sugar Intake Comes From

Knowing the facts about carbohydrates and insulin response gives you a good idea of which carbs to eat and which to stay away from. This section goes into more detail about the sugar content of common foods and ways you can identify hidden sources of sugar from food labels (find more on successfully deciphering food labels in Chapter 6).

A good rule to keep in mind is to stay away from any prepared food that has more than 5 grams of sugar per 100-gram or 100-millilitre serving. That's a decent benchmark for evaluating the overall 'sugariness' of a food.

When you start paying attention to the nutrition facts of some common foods, you may very well be surprised that foods generally considered to be healthy — such as dried fruit, vitamin water, barbeque sauce, fruit yoghurts, 100-per-cent fruit juice — often have far more sugar than things you consider dessert!

Picking out obvious sources of sugar

When considering foods to stay away from, the obvious sugary treats are the easiest to identify:

- Lollies (yes, that means milk chocolate)
- Biscuits, doughnuts, scones and other sugary baked goods
- Sugared beverages like cordials, soft drinks, sports waters, energy drinks, sweet tea and flavoured milk
- Sweetened breakfast cereals

When you investigate the labels of the foods in your pantry and refrigerator, some of the common sources of sugar will be obvious — anything that says *sugar* or *syrup* is a dead giveaway. And that means give it away!

You can read all about cleaning out and restocking your kitchen in Chapter 6.

Uncovering hidden sources of sugar

Many foods that are generally considered healthy are actually quite high in sugar content. That doesn't mean that they don't have nutritional value, but it does mean that you have to be aware of how much sugar they contain. Orange juice isn't bad for you, for example, but it does have a lot of sugar and a lot of calories in one small glass. So drink it sparingly — or just eat an orange!

Here are some common foods, drinks and condiments with a sugar content that may surprise you:

- **Bottled teas:** Tea is good for you, right? Yes, but unless you make it yourself, it may be packed with sugar and other unhealthy ingredients. A 500-millilitre bottle of commercially available ice tea has . . . wait for it . . . 31 grams of sugar!
- **Children's drinks:** The average 250-millilitre juice box or popper many school kids have in their packed lunch includes 26 grams of sugar.

✔ **'Healthy' smoothies:** The juice you may pick up from your local fresh juice and smoothie chain may contain up to 90 grams of sugar!

✔ **Dried fruit:** A handful of dried fruit — or approximately 100 grams — equals 40.5 grams of sugar. Yikes! That's about 10 teaspoons of sugar.

✔ **Energy bars and muesli bars:** Several of the best-selling energy bars are nothing more than glorified sweets. Just because it has a picture of oats or an athlete on the wrapper doesn't mean it's a high-quality snack.

✔ **Sports or energy drinks:** Most energy drinks consist of caffeine, sugar and a high dose of B-vitamins to give you a buzz for an hour or two. They not only spike your insulin levels but also ensure the post-sugar crash afterward.

✔ **Fruit juice:** A 250-millilitre glass of 100-per-cent orange juice has 25 grams of sugar. Many other so-called fruit juices (or 'fruit drinks') are only around 25-per-cent juice, with the rest being high-fructose corn syrup or another sweetener (along with artificial colour, artificial flavour and preservatives).

✔ **Condiments and sauces:** Prepared sweet chilli sauces often contain around 14 grams of sugar in a 20-millilitre serve. A takeaway sandwich with loads of sauce also has loads of sugar. When eating out, don't be afraid to request items without sauces. Learn to love mustard!

✔ **Yoghurts:** Some small tubs of Australia's and New Zealand's most popular yoghurt brands have around 28 grams of sugar in their 'lite', low-in-fat fruit yoghurts.

✔ **Muesli:** Dried fruit in some of the healthiest looking muesli can make the sugar content soar. Some options can contain up to eight teaspoons of sugar in a small 40-gram serve.

✔ **Fast-food breakfast:** Just one slice of raisin toast from a cafe or fast-food venue can have 17 grams of sugar.

✔ **Salad dressing:** Fat-free salad dressings are frequently made mostly of sugar and artificial ingredients. Use organic olive oil and vinegar or lemon instead.

Spotting other names for sugar and sweeteners

Not everything that is sugar uses that specific word in the list of ingredients. Here's a reference list of some other names for sugar that you may not recognise:

Agave nectar	Fruit juice concentrate
Agave syrup	Glucose
Barley malt	Glucose solids
Beet sugar	Golden sugar
Brown rice solids	Golden syrup
Brown sugar	Grape juice concentrate
Buttered syrup	Grape sugar
Cane juice	High-fructose corn syrup
Cane juice crystals	Honey*
Cane sugar	Invert sugar
Carob syrup	Lactose
Coconut sugar*	Malt
Confectioners' sugar	Maltodextrin
Corn sugar	Maltose
Corn sweetener	Maple syrup*
Corn syrup	Molasses*
Corn syrup solids	Palm sugar
Crystallised fructose	Raw sugar
Date sugar*	Refiners' syrup
Dextran	Sorbitol
Dextrose	Sorghum syrup
Diastase	Sucanat
Diastatic malt	Sucrose
Evaporated cane juice	Turbinado sugar
Fructose	Treacle
Fruit juice	Xylitol

After you have fully transitioned into your new eating lifestyle, these forms of sweeteners may be used in extreme moderation in an option as close to natural as possible.

Considering Gluten-Free Eating

Gluten is a plant protein found in wheat, rye and barley. People trying to reduce their carbohydrate intake often also attempt to reduce gluten consumption because eliminating gluten can potentially eliminate a lot of junk food and bread from the diet. Some people have a confirmed sensitivity or allergy to gluten and cut it out of their diets to avoid the side effects. Just remember that gluten-free does not mean sugar-free!

Why are so many people sensitive to gluten? These grains are a relatively new addition to the human diet (only added about 10,000 years or so ago), so some scientists theorise that humans haven't yet adapted to digesting this type of food. Enough people exhibit a food sensitivity to gluten that it — along with dairy, nuts and GMO soy — has become one of the most common food sensitivities today. You don't have to be diagnosed with coeliac disease to have gluten intolerance.

Gluten sensitivity doesn't result in anaphylactic shock like some severe food allergies can, but it can cause long-term damage if ignored. Continued consumption of gluten by a gluten-sensitive person can lead to *coeliac disease* (sometimes referred to as *coeliac sprue*), in which gluten damages the intestines, leading to severe nutrient absorption problems and nutritional deficiencies.

 Oats don't contain gluten, but they do contain *peptide sequences* that are very similar to wheat gluten. Oats often cause symptoms in coeliac patients similar to wheat, and so we include oats in the list of foods for gluten-sensitive individuals to avoid. In addition, though oats themselves are gluten-free, they can be contaminated with gluten from other grains during distribution and processing (most oats are milled and stored in the same facilities as wheat).

Common symptoms of gluten sensitivity are

- Bloating, cramping and flatulence
- Chronic fatigue
- Diarrhoea or constipation
- Indigestion
- Joint pain
- Mouth sores
- Skin rashes
- Ulcers

Humans don't need gluten to stay healthy, so some nutritionists suggest that everyone avoid gluten, even those who aren't exhibiting any symptoms of gluten sensitivity. That doesn't make much sense to us, because avoiding all gluten can be a difficult lifestyle choice, so our suggestion is that you try eating gluten-free only if you fit any of these criteria:

- ✔ You have a confirmed gluten sensitivity or intolerance.

- ✔ You suffer from an autoimmune disorder like eczema, thyroid issues, fibromyalgia, IBS, lupus or rheumatoid arthritis.

- ✔ You've tried eating gluten-free for a few weeks, and you notice that you feel a lot better if you don't eat it.

If you've been diagnosed with coeliac disease or non-coeliac gluten sensitivity, removing gluten from your diet is very important. Cheating a little here and there may seem harmless, but it can permanently damage your intestines over time and lead to other serious problems like nutrient malabsorption, osteoporosis, depression and even intestinal cancer.

Avoiding gluten can be tricky because many common foods have ingredients that may be sources of gluten that aren't obvious. In addition to eliminating wheat, barley, rye and some oats from your diet, be aware that the following foods potentially contain gluten:

- ✔ Beer and spirits

- ✔ Stock cubes

- ✔ Lollies (sometimes dusted with wheat flour)

- ✔ Canned soups

- ✔ Cheese spreads or other processed cheese foods (why would you eat this anyway?)

- ✔ Chocolate (sometimes contains malt flavouring from barley)

- ✔ Cold meats and sausages (may have gluten from cereal fillers)

- ✔ Pre-made, processed dips

- ✔ Gravy and sauces (may have gluten in the thickening agents and liquid base)

- ✔ Dry-roasted nuts and honey-roasted nuts

- ✔ Flavoured potato chips, hot chips or other fried foods in restaurants (often coated with flour)

- ✔ Instant coffee (a cereal product is sometimes included in the formula)

- ✔ Lip balms and lipsticks

✔ Many ice creams and frozen yoghurt products

✔ Mayonnaise (ingredients that are used as thickeners may contain gluten)

✔ Precooked hams and turkeys from commercial suppliers (often basted with wheat starch and sugar)

✔ Some toothpastes

✔ Sour cream (may contain modified food starch)

 Australia and New Zealand have strict food labelling requirements, and all grains containing gluten must always be listed on the food label. If you're gluten-sensitive, you can find more thorough food information on websites like www.gfoverflow.com, www.gluten.net, www.projectallergy.com and Coeliac Australia www.coeliac.org.au. And for a complete overview of life without gluten, check out *Living Gluten-Free For Dummies* by Danna Korn and Margaret Clough (published by Wiley Australia).

Steering Clear of Artificial Sweeteners

As we guide you through your quest to reduce sugar intake, we'd be remiss if we didn't report some research about the long-term health dangers of artificial sweeteners. Much of the available research has been done with animals instead of humans, so we invite you to do your own research and draw your own conclusions. We recommend using unbleached stevia if you need to use an artificial sweetener. You may need to use this during your transition to a lower sugar way of life. But just remember — any sweetener, natural or artificial, will fuel sugar cravings.

How chemical sweeteners work

Artificial sweeteners work by causing neuro-excitation in a part of the brain that causes people to perceive a sweet taste. The danger is that these chemical sweeteners overstimulate the neurons to the point where they basically self-destruct. A recent study published in the *Yale Journal of Biology and Medicine* noted another potential danger is that artificial sweeteners may actually put weight on your body due to the sweet taste setting off a chain of physiological responses and sugar cravings.

 MSG and aspartame are especially dangerous for babies (both in and out of the womb) because infants' brains aren't yet protected by the blood–brain barrier. A possible explanation for the enormous rise of autism in American children is the mothers' use of these chemicals while pregnant (and the prevalence of these chemicals in processed food for babies and toddlers). If you're pregnant or have small children, we encourage you to investigate the research on artificial sweeteners in such journals as the *Journal of Child Neurology, Biomedica Biochimica Acta*, the *International Journal of Neuroscience*, and the *Journal of Neurochemistry*.

Monosodium glutamate (MSG)

Most folks are aware that MSG is bad news. Here's why:

- ✔ **Brain damage:** Excessive glutamate in the brain kills glutamate receptors and the neurons connected to them. This has huge implications for Alzheimer's and Parkinson's diseases.

- ✔ **Hypothalamus damage:** The hypothalamus controls other endocrine glands like the thyroid and adrenal glands.

- ✔ **Increased appetite:** The pro-MSG lobbying website (www.msgfacts.com) used to boast that one of the benefits of MSG for food manufacturers was that it caused people to eat more of their products.

- ✔ **Retinal cell damage:** MSG has been proven to cause retinal lesions.

- ✔ **Weight gain:** MSG increases the amount of insulin that the pancreas produces and causes leptin resistance. One of the standard laboratory practices to create obese mice and rats is to inject them with MSG. They're even referred to as *monosodium-glutamate-obese rats* in the research reports!

 Australia and New Zealand Food Standards state that a packaged food must declare the presence of MSG, or any other flavour enhancers, on its label, followed by the name and number. Unfortunately, to many people these names and numbers mean nothing. Here is what you need to look out for:

- ✔ 620 L: Glutamic acid

- ✔ 621: Monosodium glutamate

- ✔ 622: Monopotassium glutamate

- ✔ 623: Calcium glutamate

- ✔ 624: Monoammonium glutamate

- ✔ 625: Magnesium glutamate

- ✔ 627: Disodium guanylate

- ✔ 631: Disodium inosinate

- ✔ 635: Disodium ribonucleotides

Restaurants and cafés aren't yet required to declare the presence of these additives. If you believe you're sensitive to them, you should ask if they're being used — the owner, chef or manager should be able to tell you whether this is the case.

Some of the following products may have MSG in their ingredient list, so always read the label:

- Hydrolysed oat flour
- Hydrolysed vegetable protein
- Malt flavouring
- Natural beef (or chicken) flavouring
- Natural flavouring
- Plant protein extract
- Sodium caseinate
- Spices
- Textured vegetable protein
- Yeast extract

Aspartame (NutraSweet or Equal)

Aspartame is an artificial sweetener that was discovered by accident in 1965. Aspartame is composed of two amino acids (aspartic acid and phenylalanine) and is 200 times as sweet as table sugar. Commonly labelled as NutraSweet and Equal, it is often found in diet soft drinks, sugar-free chewing gum, and sugar-free mixes like puddings and yoghurts. Although it's nearly calorie-free, ingesting large amounts of aspartame may have some dangerous effects:

- **Brain damage:** Like MSG, aspartame kills glutamate receptors and the neurons connected to them.

- **Increased appetite:** Aspartame suppresses the production of *serotonin*, one of the neurotransmitters that make you feel full and satisfied. When your serotonin levels aren't allowed to rise as they normally do when you eat, you crave more and more food.

✓ **Methanol (wood alcohol):** Aspartame is 10 per cent methanol, which, according to the European Journal of Clinical Nutrition, 'can give rise to formaldehyde, diketopiperazine [a carcinogen], and a number of other highly toxic derivatives'.

Sucralose (Splenda)

The good news about sucralose is that it doesn't cross the blood–brain barrier, so it shouldn't cause brain damage. The bad news is that Splenda, the most common sucralose sweetener, is a *chlorocarbon*, which is a known carcinogen (and is used as a pesticide too). Chlorocarbons have long been known for causing organ, genetic and reproductive damage.

The testing of sucralose reveals that it can cause up to 40 per cent shrinkage of the *thymus*, a gland that's vital to your immune system.

In animal studies, Splenda reduces the amount of good bacteria in the intestines by 50 per cent, acidifies the intestines and contributes to increases in body weight. It also affects the P-glycoprotein in the body in such a way that certain medications (chemotherapy, AIDS treatment and drugs for heart conditions) may be rejected by shunting them back into the intestines rather than absorbing them into the body as intended.

What should you do?

Don't eat or drink products with these chemicals (or their hidden pseudonyms) on the label. If it sounds like junk when you're reading the nutritional panel, it usually is.

Proper nutrition may help protect your brain. The vitamin E and selenium in raw seeds and nuts and the *anthocyanins* in grapes and berries can play a protective role. Good research also exists on the neuroprotective effects of omega-3 fatty acids from fish and supplemental acetyl l-carnitine.

If you must eat or drink something with MSG or an artificial sweetener, make sure you have some good carbohydrates (logs) in your system. The damage that these chemicals cause to your brain is much worse when your glucose levels are low. One of the worst things you can do to your brain is drink a diet soft drink on an empty stomach!

Chapter 4

How Sugar Contributes to Chronic Health Problems

*F*rom a physiology standpoint, processed sugars like table sugar and high-fructose corn syrup are broken down in the digestive system and are dealt with somewhat like other carbohydrates from vegetables, fruits and grains. But the health problems from processed sugars stem from the fact that people get overloaded with far too much sugar and, worse, processed sugars lack the nutrients naturally found in plant carbohydrates — vitamins, minerals, fibre, antioxidants and protein.

Eating refined sugars loads you up on calories and triggers a gigantic release of insulin, sometimes without adding a single valuable nutrient or a lone gram of fibre or protein. All those empty calories add up, making sugar consumption one of the primary causes of obesity and serious health concerns throughout much of the world.

High sugar intake has been proven to lower the effectiveness of your immune system. It also promotes inflammation and produces damaging by-products. Sugar disrupts the natural energy production of the body's adrenal cortex, so it can lead to chronic fatigue and depression.

So, if obesity, diabetes, fatigue, metabolic syndrome, osteoporosis and inflammatory diseases aren't enough reasons to change your eating habits, think about the ramifications of a self-inflicted illness on your family and loved ones. You can read about all these health problems — and quite a few more — in this chapter.

Sugar Highs: Looking at Escalating Health Problems

Sugar consumption worldwide has skyrocketed in recent decades, and this increase has resulted in a corresponding rise in obesity, diabetes and other health problems. The low-fat craze in the 1990s exacerbated the sugar overload in our food supply. People wanting to do the 'right thing' nutritionally went from low-fat to high carbs within a decade. When fat is removed from food, it becomes tasteless, so manufacturers added lots of sugar and salt to make up for the missing flavour. Sugar doesn't have any fat, so manufacturers can still put '100 per cent fat-free' labels on a two-kilogram bag of sugar.

The American Heart Association (AHA) recommends limiting the amount of added sugars you consume daily. For women, they recommend no more than six teaspoons of added sugar and, for men, nine teaspoons. In Australia and New Zealand, no authority has given such easy-to-use guidelines, so you can rely on the AHA statistics. The AHA recommendations focus on all added sugars, without singling out any particular types such as high-fructose corn syrup.

An epidemic of diabetes is occurring in Australia and New Zealand, as it is in the rest of the world. Over one million Australians have diabetes and at least 85 per cent of these have type 2 diabetes, which is largely preventable. The disease shortens life expectancy by up to five years and costs the community nearly $14.6 billion per year, with Diabetes Australia predicting costs will double to $30 billion in 12 years if preventative approaches aren't adopted.

Society needs to change its approach to diabetes, and to change it quickly. People need to begin looking at the *prevention* of diabetes rather than its management. In a study published in the journal *Diabetologia*, of the nearly 2,500 diabetes-related trials looked at, 75 per cent emphasised diabetes treatment, while only 10 per cent examined preventive measures. Prevention is better than management — and you can begin with what you're placing in your mouth at every meal and every snack.

Seeing the Psychological Ramifications of Sugar

Sugar is a food, but it has drug-like effects on your brain. Sugar triggers the pleasure centre of your brain just like alcohol and cocaine, and it can become just as addictive. Sugar affects the chemistry of both your body and your brain, and sugar addicts commonly struggle with depression, anxiety or both.

Depression

The primary cause of depression is a problem with the hormone *serotonin*, which is a substance that makes people feel happy and satisfied. Serotonin also converts to *melatonin* in healthy individuals, which assists in a good night's sleep. Most serotonin is produced in the gut. Many things affect the body's production of serotonin, including stress, nutrition and sleep.

Chronic overconsumption of sugar causes the body to produce less serotonin on its own because it starts relying on the external supply from your sugary diet. This lack of natural serotonin production can cause depression and create a situation where you need sugar to feel good, because you're producing less serotonin without it.

Too much sugar is 'carbicide' (or death by carbs) to your happiness for other reasons as well:

✔ Excess sugar contributes to insulin and leptin resistance and plays havoc with your mental health.

✔ Too much sugar suppresses *brain derived neurotropic factor* (BDNF), a growth hormone that nurtures healthy brain neurons. BDNF is low in people with depression and schizophrenia.

✔ Added sugars can trigger chemical reactions in your body that promote inflammation. Inflammation disrupts the normal functioning of your immune system and is linked to depression.

To maintain a normal level of endorphins in the brain, the sugar abuser must eat more sugar and carbohydrates to relieve the state of depression and maintain a normal mood level. This causes a vicious cycle of addiction. Interestingly, this is exactly the same cycle that develops with excessive alcohol intake. Alcohol abuse, like sugar abuse, causes many of the endorphin sites to shut down, so to get the feel-good effects normally given by endorphins, the alcoholic must continue to drink alcohol instead.

Additionally, B-vitamins (especially B3, B6 and folic acid), which are essential for the production of serotonin, are used up to metabolise all that sugar, leaving less for the production of serotonin and increasing energy levels, and other important uses.

Excess *fructose* (a simple sugar we describe in Chapter 3) can exacerbate depression. Research has shown that people who have trouble metabolising fructose (up to half the population) have lower levels of *tryptophan* (a serotonin precursor). They also have lower serum zinc and folic acid levels, both of which are associated with depression. Women already have lower serum levels of tryptophan than men do (which is likely part of the reason why women are more vulnerable to depression), so depleting tryptophan in the diet with fructose may lead to even lower levels, and thus depression.

Statistically, women are more prone to clinical depression than men for several reasons, one being oestrogen. Oestrogen activates an enzyme called *hepatic tryptophan 2, 3 dioxygenase* (don't worry; there won't be a quiz) that shifts the metabolism of tryptophan from making serotonin (the happy hormone) to making kynurenic acid (a substance that hinders brain function). Maybe that's why women get 'baby brain' or severe mood swings when oestrogen levels rise during pregnancy or decrease during menopause.

Blood sugar spikes actually destabilise the brain through a harmful process called glycation. *Glycation* is the chemical process in the body whereby sugars, proteins and certain fats become tangled together, making all manner of body tissues stiff and inflexible — including the brain. Glycation causes damage in the body that induces rapid ageing effects (see the 'Wrinkles' section later in the chapter) and physically shrinks your brain tissue.

According to the Mayo Clinic, people with depression often have low blood levels of the essential fats *eicosapentaenoic acid* (EPA) and *docosahexaenoic acid* (DHA). Good sources of these essential nutrients are chia seeds, ground linseeds and cold-water fish like salmon (fresh or canned), gemfish, blue eye trevalla, blue mackerel, oysters, sardines, trout and tuna, and distilled fish oil capsules (see Chapter 5 for more information about helpful nutrition supplements). Sugar addicts struggling with depression may want to consider adding extra sources of these important fats to their diet.

Anxiety

Sugar addicts commonly suffer from anxiety. Sugar abuse produces a blood-sugar roller-coaster that can trigger anxiety attacks. When blood sugar levels crash, your brain gets desperate for food, and your body can become shaky, weak, confused and anxious. If you find yourself at midmorning feeling like this, ask yourself whether you had a proper breakfast. Do the feelings happen to you again in the afternoon? What kind of nourishment have you fed yourself for lunch? As blood sugar levels plummet, the brain reacts by sending out a panicked adrenaline alarm, leading to severe anxiety. People who are prone to anxiety attacks generally walk around in a state of heightened stress anyway, so it doesn't take much to push them over the edge — a sugar crash is often just the ticket.

Another way that sugar can cause an anxiety attack is by causing lactic acid to build up in the bloodstream. *Lactic acid* is the final product in the breakdown of blood sugar (glucose) when a lack of oxygen is experienced. If you're prone to anxiety, a build-up of carbon dioxide and lactic acid in the blood causes a pH change in your brain that signals your amygdala to trigger feelings of anxiety and fear.

Adrenaline junkies often report that they need caffeine or sugar to jump-start their energy in the morning. To calm yourself down and gradually coax your adrenal glands back into normal functioning, start weaning yourself off sugar and coffee, and try green tea instead. Green tea contains less caffeine than coffee and high amounts of the amino acid *l-theanine,* which can help you stay calm and focused. A good-quality green tea is also high in antioxidants. Licorice tea is another smart choice — it's naturally sweet and helps improve your adrenal function.

Dealing with Medical Risks and Problems

The estimated annual health-care costs of obesity, diabetes, depression, cancer and metabolic syndrome combined are in the hundreds of millions of dollars in Australia alone. Costs in New Zealand are also extremely high.

Poor nutrition (with sugar abuse leading the way) causes a long list of medical problems, which are mostly preventable through a healthy lifestyle and a high-quality diet. We cover many of these medical problems in the following sections.

Obesity

The Centres for Disease Control and Prevention report that obesity has overtaken cigarette smoking for the number one spot on the list of health-care costs.

Overconsumption of sugar causes obesity in two primary ways: excess calories and excess *insulin* (the hormone that shuttles sugar from the blood into cells).

Excess calories

Sugar contains no nutrients to speak of, only calories. Because it lacks fibre and nutrients, sugar bypasses your body's natural leptin response (*leptin* is the hormone that signals your brain that you have enough body fat), so even after eating hundreds of calories in sugar, you don't feel satisfied. Perhaps you always feel hungry, or know someone else who feels this way. If you eat a primarily high-carb meal, you'll be hungry again 90 minutes later.

It only takes eating 400 extra kilojoules (kJ) per day to gain 4.5 kilograms over a year! Multiply that by ten years and you may start to understand why your belts are too tight. And consuming 400 kilojoules in a quick snack is easy — it's what's contained in around four squares of chocolate, and even so-called healthy muesli bars can contain this amount of kilojoules or more. Sugary junk foods are low in nutrients and high in calories. High-sugar diets cause more sugar cravings and a strong desire for more carbohydrates. Be sure to get your carbohydrates from vegetables, which are high in nutrients and low in calories. The fibre and 'crunchy' factor help you feel full. Whole grains, seed and nuts are also high in fibre and nutrients.

Fructose (refer to Chapter 3) appears to affect leptin sensitivity more than other sugars. If you consistently overeat fructose, your brain can become insensitive to leptin — a condition known as *leptin resistance*. Unable to sense leptin, your brain lowers your metabolism to try to conserve fat stores. To replace the 'missing' body fat, your body packages up any dietary fat present in the high-fructose food and stores it as body fat. Common foods with high concentrations of fructose are fruit juice, processed cakes, biscuits, muffins and agave nectar.

Excess insulin

Eating too much sugar at one time leads to a large release of insulin to control the amount of sugar in the bloodstream. High insulin levels erroneously tell the brain that, because the system has excess insulin, your cells must be starving for glucose. In response, your brain creates cravings for carbohydrates and signals your body to store fat. Excess body fat causes insulin resistance, so obesity both *causes* and *is caused by* type 2 diabetes (see the next section for details).

In women, excess insulin also stimulates the ovaries to produce excess testosterone, which can cause infertility by preventing the ovaries from releasing an egg each month. High levels of insulin also increase the conversion of *androgens* (male hormones) to *oestrogens* (female hormones), upsetting the delicate balance between the two and having a direct effect on the formation of cystic follicles or cysts in the ovary. For this reason, women with polycystic ovary syndrome (PCOS) must control their insulin levels through diet.

Interestingly, you don't have to be fat to have high insulin levels. Michele sees female patients in her clinic with high insulin and PCOS, and refers to them as 'fat and unhealthy on the inside' — thin women who live on high sugar and have massive inflammation, oxidation and hormonal issues going on inside.

Diabetes

Several types of diabetes exist, but the diabetes epidemic relates to *type 2 diabetes*, which is caused by a diet that keeps insulin levels high. Eating too many carbohydrates (especially sugar) leads to excess insulin production and increased body fat. Large amounts of body fat and frequent high insulin levels decrease your ability to respond to your own insulin. This inability of your cells to respond to insulin is termed *insulin resistance*, and it causes your cells to 'refuse' the glucose from the blood (for more on this, see the sidebar 'Insulin: Comparing normal and impaired function'). When glucose builds up in the blood instead of going into cells, it can lead to serious problems like organ damage, nerve damage (neuropathy), blindness, hearing loss, heart disease and stroke.

High insulin levels suppress the production of two important hormones: *glucagon* and *growth hormone*. Your body secretes glucagon when your blood sugar levels are low because its job is to trigger the release of stored fuel to be burned for energy. High insulin levels shut down glucagon production, so you can't burn fat and you begin to store it.

Your body uses growth hormone for muscle repair and building new muscle tissue. Insulin resistance reduces muscle development, which keeps your metabolism slow.

Type 2 diabetes leads to a vicious catch-22 that makes weight loss more difficult and blood sugar control less reliable. High levels of insulin can lead to insulin resistance, and this means your cells are deprived of glucose and nutrients — the glucose and the nutrients can't get in to the cells without the insulin that allows the entry. Sadly, this means the cells — and so the body — are literally starving. The cells are starving for glucose and nutrients and this creates a perpetual cycle of hunger and fat storage.

Type 2 diabetes goes hand in hand with other 'lifestyle' diseases like elevated cholesterol and triglycerides, obesity and chronic stress issues. Type 2 diabetes does have some genetic risk factors but is more often lifestyle induced, meaning your children may develop type 2 diabetes due to what is being stored in the pantry and fridge. (Michele even knows a family who has a dog with type 2 diabetes!)

The good news is that you can reverse insulin resistance relatively quickly by lowering your simple carbohydrate intake and doing some basic exercise (flip to Chapter 12 for advice on exercise).

Cinnamon contains substances (*methylhydroxy chalcone* polymers, if you're a chemistry nerd) that may make insulin receptors more sensitive. Using cinnamon instead of sugar provides a sweet taste and a no-sugar alternative in the fight against type 2 diabetes.

Insulin: Comparing normal and impaired function

Insulin transports other nutrients besides glucose, including amino acids from protein and lipid molecules from fats. Insulin connects with special *insulin receptors* on cell surfaces and acts as a 'key' to open up the cells to receive nutrients. Insulin receptors are on virtually all body tissues, including muscle and fat cells. When you become insulin-resistant, your cells don't respond to insulin properly. This table compares normal insulin response with impaired insulin response:

When insulin receptors function correctly:	When you have insulin resistance:
Insulin transports glucose into cells, clearing it from the bloodstream.	Glucose isn't cleared from the bloodstream; the excess sugar damages tissues and creates inflammation.
Glucose is stored in the liver and in muscle cells as *glycogen* for fuel (ensuring you always have the ability to fuel your body).	Glucose isn't stored properly, and cells get starved for energy. The brain increases cravings for more sugar.
Insulin moves amino acids into muscles, stimulating repair and growth.	Muscles lack essential amino acids and begin to break down, rather than creating lean muscle mass.
The insulin/glucagon axis functions properly to break down fat for energy when needed.	Chronically high insulin levels shut off fat burning and stimulate fat storage.

Although chronic excess insulin production from a poor diet causes the vast majority of insulin resistance cases, insulin resistance can result from several different problems, including genetics, the shape of your insulin (preventing receptor binding), lack of an adequate number of insulin receptors, signalling problems, or glucose transporters not working properly. Whatever the specific cause, the function of insulin becomes impaired, and the same health problems occur. Reducing your carbohydrate intake helps reduce the harmful effects of insulin resistance, regardless of the genesis of your condition.

Liver disease

When you eat excess sugar, especially in the form of fructose, your body sends it to the liver, which converts the molecules into triglycerides (basically fat). The liver exports the triglycerides into the bloodstream, where they're picked up and stored as body fat. The transport system that moves triglycerides from the liver into the bloodstream can only work so fast, so if too much fructose enters the liver at once, the triglycerides accumulate inside the liver, leading to a condition called (unsurprisingly) *fatty liver* or more specifically *non-alcoholic fatty liver disease* (NAFLD).

Liver disease and cirrhosis of the liver *used* to be terms associated with an older population and alcoholics. Sadly, this is not the case anymore. A review in the *Journal of Clinical Gastroenterology* reveals that NALFD is believed to be one of the most common forms of liver disease worldwide, with its prevalence growing in proportion to the increase in obesity. Experts are concerned at how many children and young people in the developed world are being diagnosed with this disease and predict that, by 2020, NALFD will be the number one reason for liver transplants. This trend becomes even sadder when you consider NALFD is reversible with diet and exercise if you get to it before cirrhosis occurs.

In adults and children with fatty liver disease, the fat that accumulates causes inflammation and scarring of the liver. This more serious form of liver disease is called *non-alcoholic steatohepatitis*, or NASH for short. At its most severe, fatty liver disease can progress to liver failure, which means transplant or death. Given the increasing rates of this disease in people of all ages, poor eating choices is a serious issue, not a cosmetic issue! We need to be preventive with nutrition not prescriptive with medications.

Sugar and cholesterol

When you think of the word *cholesterol*, you may also immediately think of the word *fat*. However, as current medical experts and researchers focus on the detrimental effects of sugar, they're reassessing the real culprit for cholesterol issues. The preceding section on liver disease explains how sugar creates triglycerides. The body makes *very low-density lipoprotein* (VLDL) to transport these extra triglycerides. As the VLDL circulates in the blood, triglycerides are deposited and the particle gets smaller, eventually becoming a *low-density lipoprotein* (LDL), the 'bad' cholesterol. The more sugar you eat, the more harmful LDL you're left with.

That small bag of lollies, such as snakes or jelly beans, you get from the supermarket can have '99 per cent fat-free' in large print on the front of the bag. This claim is true, because sugar has no fat. A two-kilogram bag of lollies can make the same claim, yet when this sugar is ingested in excess, it becomes fat in the form of triglycerides.

High insulin levels (from high carbohydrate intake) also raise cholesterol production in the body by stimulating the cholesterol-producing enzyme *HMG-CoA reductase*.

High sugar consumption lowers *high-density lipoprotein* (HDL), the 'good' cholesterol that acts as a vacuum cleaner and removes cholesterol from the arterial walls. Low HDL is one of the hallmarks of metabolic syndrome (see the next section). The more sugar you eat, the lower your good HDL and the higher your bad LDL and triglycerides.

Refined sugar contains no fibre, but vegetables, whole grains and fruits do! Dietary fibre sweeps cholesterol out of the body before it can be absorbed, keeping your arteries clear of build-up that would otherwise turn into dangerous plaque on the arterial walls. Try to eat at least 30 grams of dietary fibre each day.

Metabolic syndrome

Metabolic syndrome (also known as *syndrome X*) is a term used to describe the inevitable results of the typical high-sugar diet: Abdominal fat, elevated triglycerides, high blood pressure and high blood sugar levels.

Metabolic syndrome should be renamed 'excess carbohydrate sickness' because that's really what it is. Stop eating so many carbohydrates and your 'syndrome' will disappear!

With a high-carbohydrate diet, the insulin receptors on the cells become less and less sensitive. Because the sugar can no longer enter the cells like it's supposed to, it gets stored as fat instead. Think of the process like a slippery dip that allows glucose to come in and fuel and nourish your cell. When that insulin receptor gets abused from excess sugar, it doesn't allow the glucose to slide into the cell any longer. Your cells are literally starving for glucose and nutrients and you're actually feeling starving all the time! Eating a high-sugar diet over time turns your body into a fat-storing factory — you can take in thousands of calories each day, but little of it supplies lean tissue. Your muscle content drops (which lowers your metabolism), while fat storage becomes more and more efficient. All that body fat increases inflammation, and the insulin resistance refuses to let your body think you've had enough food.

The only way to reverse this downward spiral is to reduce your carbohydrate intake and to commit to exercise a few times per week (see Chapter 12 for exercise advice).

Figure 4-1 shows the current clinical definition of metabolic syndrome set by the International Diabetes Federation at the time of writing.

Central obesity	Waist circumference ≥ 94 centimetres for men, ≥ 80 centimetres for women; there are slightly different values for Asian ethnicities
Plus at least two of the following:	
Elevated triglycerides	≥ 150 milligrams/deciliter, or to be under treatment for elevated triglycerides
Reduced HDL (good) cholesterol	< 40 milligrams/deciliter for men, < 50 milligrams/deciliter for women, or to be under treatment for low HDL cholesterol
Elevated blood pressure	Systolic ≥ 130, diastolic ≥ 85, or to be under treatment for hypertension
Elevated fasting plasma glucose levels	≥ 100 milligrams/deciliter, or previous diagnosis of type 2 diabetes

Figure 4-1: Defining metabolic syndrome.

Illustration by Wiley, Composition Services Graphics

Hypothyroid disease

Health experts estimate that 10 per cent of Australians and New Zealanders are diagnosed with thyroid disorder from abnormal pathology results, but the true figures are much higher. In Michele's clinic, she sees one out of four women over the age of 40 with subclinical thyroid conditions. Your thyroid function is strongly affected by diet, genetics, toxins and stress.

After you eat too much sugar, you get a large rush of sugar into the bloodstream. This forces your pancreas to release a mountain of insulin that leads to a corresponding low-blood-sugar crash shortly afterward. (Remember — what goes up eventually comes down.) Low blood sugar not only stimulates more cravings but also triggers a release of the stress hormone *cortisol*, and its job is to break down carbohydrates stored in the muscles to bring blood sugar levels back up to normal. Repeated cortisol releases from episodes of low blood sugar suppress the function of the *pituitary gland*, and without proper pituitary function, your thyroid doesn't function properly.

Low thyroid function and excess sugar form a catch-22: Low thyroid function slows insulin's clearing of glucose from the blood, and high sugar levels slow thyroid output. When you're *hypothyroid*, your cells aren't very sensitive to glucose, and because your cells don't get the glucose they need, your adrenal glands release cortisol to increase the amount of glucose available to them. As long as you keep yourself on the sugar-binge-then-crash roller-coaster, your thyroid can't work properly and your adrenal glands are exhausted.

Another common source of thyroid issues is *Hashimoto's thyroiditis*, an autoimmune condition where the body makes antibodies against its own thyroid tissue. Studies have shown that the insulin spikes caused by high sugar intake increase the destruction of the thyroid gland in people with Hashimoto's disease.

Chronic fatigue

Chronic stress activates the adrenal glands to produce stress hormones like cortisol and epinephrine. Overproduction of these hormones drops your blood sugar because stress hormones make you burn circulating blood sugar for energy instead of body fat. When blood sugar drops, your brain turns on the sugar cravings to replace the burned-off sugar.

When you're stressed all the time, your adrenal glands can't keep up with the constant workload, so they lose their ability to continue churning out enough hormones to keep glucose in your system. The result is a consistent underproduction of cortisol, which in turn yields low blood sugar, chronic fatigue and more sugar cravings.

Chronic fatigue doesn't come just from stress; it comes from excess sugar too. Insulin resistance causes the cells to refuse the action of insulin trying to bring sugar into cells to be burned for energy. The result is more sugar circulating in the bloodstream and less sugar available to be metabolised for energy. This makes you tired — unspeakably tired, no matter how much you sleep. Cells are unable to take up the glucose they require, and muscles can't restock their fuel supplies of glycogen. The whole system begins to shut down and becomes an exhausted, non-functional mess.

Chronic fatigue is one of the most difficult conditions for the medical community to treat. Time and time again patients with chronic fatigue syndrome tell us how cutting back on sugar has delivered them back their old 'pep', when nothing else seemed to work.

Fibromyalgia

Fibromyalgia is one of the terms given to the condition of chronic, widespread musculoskeletal pain and fatigue. Emotional stress coupled with inflammation from too much sugar causes the nervous system to remain in an overactive state, keeping muscles 'turned on' when they shouldn't be. This causes muscles to go into tight, spastic knots that reduce circulation. As a result of the decrease in blood flow, muscles don't get the oxygen they need, and metabolic waste products start to build up. This activates nerves in the area, causing pain and constant fatigue.

Sugar damages cells through a process called *glycation* that causes muscle tissue and fascia to become stiffer and thicker. This makes chronic pain conditions worse because the inflexible tissue becomes extremely sensitive to touch and movement.

If you have chronic pain, always remember that your body chemistry is affected by your emotions too! Every single thought and emotion you have triggers certain chemical reactions throughout your body. If you truly believe that you're healthy and powerful, your body chemistry moves toward that reality. If you consistently obsess over how bad you feel or you believe that something is always wrong with you and that you'll never be well, your sickness becomes more deeply rooted in your physiology. Careful what you tell yourself — your brain is listening! Consider nourishing yourself with things other than food — try massage, meditation or easy yoga classes.

Irritable bowel syndrome

Not surprisingly, your digestive system is one of the first body systems to be affected by your diet. Consistent consumption of fast food, chemicals and high-sugar food creates a continuous state of inflammation in the gut. High sugar consumption elevates blood acid levels and increases levels of inflammatory markers like *C-reactive protein* and *homocysteine*, and this consistent inflammation can lead to a chronic irritation of the digestive system known as *irritable bowel syndrome* (IBS).

If you're under constant stress, be it emotional stress or physical stress from inflammation, your nervous system stays overstimulated, which results in a decrease in production of digestive enzymes and less movement of the bowels, which makes the irritable bowel condition worse.

If you have a fructose absorption problem (up to half of the population does), the *GLUT5 transporter* in the small intestine doesn't take up fructose as efficiently as it could. That means a lot of undigested fructose travels down to the colon, feeding the bacteria there and leading to bloating, cramping and diarrhoea — all symptoms of irritable bowel syndrome. If you have IBS, avoid consuming too much fructose at one time.

An acidic, high-sugar diet creates an environment in the intestines that creates an imbalance or decrease in the beneficial bacteria (the *intestinal flora*) that colonise the gut. This makes way for harmful organisms to take hold, including parasites, infectious bacteria and yeast (see the next section). Disrupting the intestinal flora adds to bowel irritation by compromising both digestion and immunity.

Immune system impairment

Research clearly shows that ingesting large amounts of sugar results in a significant decrease in the ability of the immune system to engulf bacteria. This effect occurs rapidly after eating sugar and lasts for several hours afterwards. If you eat sugary foods several times per day, you're keeping your immune system in a depressed state almost constantly!

A high-sugar diet destroys the *intestinal flora* — the beneficial bacteria that are crucial to digestion and the immune system's proper functioning. Transitioning to a low-sugar, high-vegetable diet and using a probiotic supplement (see Chapter 5) can help re-establish the intestinal flora and restore your immune system back to normal function. Two common results of faulty immune system function are detailed in the following sections.

Yeast infections

Vaginal yeast infections are usually caused by an overgrowth of *Candida albicans,* a fungus normally found in only tiny amounts in dark, damp nooks and crannies of the body. Your immune system usually keeps the amount of *Candida* in check, but when your immune system is compromised, overgrowths aren't uncommon. For women, these nasty infections are often one of the first signs of high insulin levels.

Ingesting sugar lowers your immune response almost immediately. A high-sugar diet also reduces the amount of beneficial bacteria in the intestines (as does antibiotic use), further weakening the immune system.

Yeast feeds on sugar, and it grows best in an acidic environment. A high-sugar diet gives it both!

Autoimmune disorders

Your body is under a constant barrage of attacks from not only bacteria and viruses but also pollution, pesticides, radiation, chemicals, carcinogens, metal poisoning, and other exposures both seen and unseen. Your immune system is strongly affected by your diet, your lifestyle, your environment and your stress level.

One of the theories of the genesis of autoimmune diseases is that, over time, chronic stress and poor diet cause cells to become less efficient at eliminating waste products and toxins. Eventually, these waste products and toxins incorporate themselves into your cell membranes, causing your immune system to identify such cells as being damaged or foreign. At that point, your immune system tags these diseased cells with antibodies and starts attacking them.

High blood sugar levels damage your body's tissues and trigger an inflammatory response. Chronic inflammation is the hallmark of autoimmune disorders because it keeps the immune system on overdrive.

In addition to causing inflammation, overconsumption of sugar (especially fructose) causes overgrowth of bacteria and yeast in the large intestine, which keeps the immune system on overdrive in an attempt to quell the continuous infestation.

Bone loss and tooth decay

Excess sugar has a negative effect on all your tissues, including your bones and teeth. This section explains how sugar contributes to problems with bone density and tooth decay.

Osteoporosis and osteopenia

Osteoporosis (and its precursor, *osteopenia*) are conditions that describe varying degrees of bone loss (also referred to as *thinning of the bones*). Bone loss occurs when your body breaks down bone tissue faster than it makes new bone. When your bones are too thin, you're at risk of dangerous and debilitating fractures — one in five hip fracture patients dies within a year of their injury! Without getting too technical, sugar contributes to osteoporosis by raising the acidity of the blood, requiring your body to restore its acid/alkaline balance by breaking down bone tissue to flood the blood with calcium to neutralise the excess acid.

After overdosing on sugar, the resulting sugar crash causes a significant increase in your cortisol levels. Long-term elevation of cortisol can cause severe bone loss.

Diets high in grains can promote bone density problems too, because the *phytic acid* in grains binds to calcium and other minerals, limiting absorption. For strong bones, eat your veggies, decrease the bread, and stay away from the sweets!

Tooth decay and bad breath

Tooth decay starts when you eat sugar and bacteria metabolise the carbohydrates to form acids that dissolve tooth enamel. Bacteria multiply rapidly in the wet, sugary environment of the addict's mouth, and a decayed tooth soon results.

Research shows that frequent consumption of sugar, particularly when eaten alone between meals, promotes tooth decay. Sugars and starches are less cavity-producing when ingested along with protein, fat and water. So if you want to keep your teeth healthy, don't snack on sugar.

The bacteria that live off the sugar stuck to your tooth enamel produce smelly by-products that can give you bad breath. These bacteria can cause infection and inflammation of the gums too.

Wrinkles

Sugar causes *glycation* of tissues in the body, making them stiffer and less elastic. Sugar in your system attaches to proteins to form harmful new molecules called *advanced glycation end products* (or, ironically, AGEs for short). The more sugar you eat, the more AGEs you develop.

Glycated tissue yields rapid ageing effects, including loss of elasticity of the skin (wrinkles) and cataracts. AGEs deactivate your body's natural antioxidant enzymes, leaving your skin more vulnerable to sun damage.

In addition to cutting back on the amount of sugar you eat, look for 'skin food' — that is, food that's rich in vitamin C and antioxidants, such as fresh vegetables and lemons or limes. Vitamin C assists in the formation of collagen, which is one of the keys to keeping wrinkles at bay.

Sleep deprivation

Figuring out whether sleep deprivation comes before or after sugar addiction can be hard, but one thing is for sure — the cycle can be difficult to get out of. Medical science studies show sleep deprivation leads to excess weight gain, poor immunity, stressed adrenals and poor cognitive function.

Sugar bingers who snack on sweet treats after dinner are really setting themselves up for the 'tired but wired' syndrome we see in our clinics in at least 75 per cent of our patients, regardless of their age. Taking in even a few biscuits or a yoghurt with hidden sugars can spike your blood glucose, giving you the 'wired' feeling even though your body is saying it's time for bed. Then, after you finally do fall asleep, the sugar roller-coaster continues to roll — this time, on the downwards slope. Often patients say they wake at 2 am and perhaps have to go to the toilet or feel hungry — some are sweaty or even feel anxious. All of these are symptoms of low blood sugar and show what can occur when blood sugar dips dramatically after a sugar spike.

Part II

Developing Your Low-Sugar Food Plan

Serving Size	Nutritional Information			Per 100g
This is the average serving size of the product as determined by the manufacturer. However, this may not be the same as the serving you have.	**SERVINGS PER PACKAGE: 3** **SERVING SIZE: 15G**	**Qty per serving**	**Qty per 100g**	100g is a useful standard to compare products eg: which is lower in fat. Use this information when choosing products.
	Energy	608kJ	405kJ	
	Protein	4.2g	2.8g	
	Fat, total — saturated	7.4g 4.5g	4.9g 3.0g	
	Carbohydrate — total — sugars	18.6g 18.6g	12.4g 12.4g	
	Sodium	90mg	60mg	

FAT	**CARBOHYDRATE**	**SODIUM (salt)**
Total This is the total amount of fat in the product. It includes the amount of fat from the three main types of fat: saturated, polyunsaturated and monounsaturated. **Saturated** Use the figure per 100g, compare similar products and pick the one with less saturated fat.	**Total** This includes both sugars and starches in food. If you are counting carbohydrates you can use this figure to work out how much carbohydrate is in the food. **Sugars** This tells you how much of the total carbohydrate is sugar. This includes 'added sugar' as well as naturally occurring sugars like lactose (milk sugar) and fructose (fruit sugar). Sugar content alone will not predict the effect of the food on your blood glucose level.	Choose, where possible, products with reduced or no added salt.

web extras

Find out key reasons why losing weight is so difficult for some people at
www.dummies.com/extras/beatingsugaraddictionau.

In this part . . .

- ✔ Create a foundation of good nutrition in order to better manage your appetite and stay craving-free.
- ✔ Take charge of managing your kilojoules and practising portion control.
- ✔ Consider adding nutrition supplements to your daily routine for health and nutrition help.
- ✔ Tap into the benefits of a sugar detox, and navigate traditional and alternative methods for dealing with sugar abuse.

Chapter 5

Creating a Sustainable Plan: The Basics of Nutrition and Portions

· ·

In This Chapter

▶ Getting enough (and the right kind of) protein, carbs, fats and water

▶ Choosing natural produce, meat, dairy, eggs and fish

▶ Watching your kilojoules and portions

▶ Fortifying your diet with the right nutrition supplements

· ·

*T*he avalanche of nutrition advice available from the media and the internet can be overwhelming. Our goal for this chapter is to deliver the facts to you as they are currently understood — without gimmicks or special 'diets' — and give you a system for designing a sensible, sustainable, low-sugar eating plan that works for you from this day forward.

This chapter talks about the basic *macronutrients* (protein, carbohydrates and fat) that you need to build your nutritional foundation, as well as the importance of water. We also discuss kilojoules and portion control and deliver an important explanation of why a kilojoule is not just a kilojoule. Another topic of discussion is nutrition supplements for improving overall health — and for reducing sugar cravings too!

We're sceptical about any fad diets or quick fixes for weight loss and wellbeing. The information delivered in this chapter (and in this book) isn't just useful for the next few weeks; it's useful for the remainder of your life!

Creating a Low-Sugar Foundation with the Big Four

Even though the focus of this book is freeing yourself from the unhealthy grip of sugar, we invite you to think on a larger scale and create a new, healthy nutrition system for yourself (and for your family, if you're feeding them too).

A nutrition foundation starts with the three *macronutrients* (protein, carbohydrates and fats) and water. These are the big four that you can't live without. The macronutrients are the components of foods that supply you with kilojoules to stay alive and with raw materials to maintain and renew your cells, muscles, organs, brain and all your other tissues.

Adopt the question 'Have I had my macros today?' as your new daily thought. Protein is for blood sugar regulation, fat is for curbing sweet cravings, and complex carbs are for energy.

Picking protein

Dietary protein is essential for maintaining the structure of your body. All the soft tissues in the body — muscles, ligaments, tendons, organs, and even skin and hair — are made of protein. Most enzymes are proteins, and your body uses proteins to catalyse almost all the reactions in living cells — so proteins control virtually every cellular process. The major neurotransmitters are proteins, and your immune cells and antibodies all have proteins attached to them. If you would like lean muscle mass, happy hormones and a strong immune system, make sure quality proteins are included in your meals.

Most of the high-quality sources of protein are sugar-free, but dairy sources of protein are often higher in carbohydrates than meat, poultry, fish and eggs. Some protein is present in grains and legumes too.

You digest protein more slowly than carbohydrates, so it slows blood sugar release and helps you feel satisfied for a longer period of time. Eating protein also boosts your metabolic rate more than eating fat or carbohydrates. If you're a sugar addict, one of the keys to success during your transition to low sugar is ensuring you have protein at each meal and even at your morning tea and afternoon tea. Why? Doing so keeps your blood sugar from spiking and dipping.

Understanding protein quality

So why are some proteins better than others? What makes a good protein? Proteins are made up of strings of *amino acids*. Nutrition scientists have identified 22 specific amino acids that are found in the human body.

These amino acids combine in different ways to synthesise proteins that the body uses for building structures and for various chemical and enzymatic processes.

Your body is very good at being able to rig stuff and pull off stunts to obtain adequate nutrients and stay alive. One of these cool skills is that your body can actually manufacture many of these 22 amino acids if it's supplied with 9 specific amino acids. These 9 amino acids are termed *essential amino acids* because the body can't manufacture them — they must be obtained through food. One of the criteria used to determine the quality of a protein is its content of essential amino acids.

If your food doesn't supply enough of even one of the essential amino acids, your body begins to break down its protein structures — muscle and organs — to obtain the missing amino acids. The human body doesn't store excess amino acids for later use, like it does with fat and carbohydrate. Amino acids must be present in the food, so it's important to try to eat a quality protein source every few hours throughout the day to avoid muscle tissue breakdown. This breakdown, by the way, is called *catabolism*, and it results in lowered metabolism and less fat-burning potential.

Finding sources of protein

The best protein sources come from animals in the form of meat, poultry, eggs, fish and dairy. Plants like soy, nuts and legumes can also supply you with some dietary protein. The following is a summary of these protein sources, in descending order of *biological value* (protein quality).

The healthiest foods come from organic, natural sources. That means you'll ideally use pasture-fed, meat, poultry and eggs, and wild-caught fish and prawns (not farmed) whenever possible. Choose organic vegetable proteins to steer clear of pesticides and genetically modified food. See the later section 'Eating Natural Foods' for details.

Getting protein from animal sources

All proteins from animal sources are complete proteins, meaning that they contain all the essential amino acids you need for creating structural and functional proteins. You can get protein from the following sources (the highest-quality sources are at the top of the list):

✔ **Whey:** Powdered, pure whey protein, which is derived from grass-fed dairy (may have up to 4 per cent lactose), scores highest in all the protein efficiency ratings and tops the list as the highest-quality protein per kilojoule. *Note:* We're talking about a 'clean' whey powder here, not a 'protein powder' concoction with words on it that you (or a trainer or nutritionist) can't decipher or pronounce. (We cover whey protein later, in the 'Adding Supplements for Health and Help' section.)

- ✓ **Eggs:** Eggs provide protein and healthy fat, along with vitamins and *carotenoids* that can reduce your risk of developing cataracts and age-related macular degeneration. Eggs also contain *choline*, a nutrient that's essential to normal cell structure and proper signalling of nerve cells. The egg white contains most of the protein, and the yolks provide the other healthy nutrients. Eggs are inexpensive compared to other proteins so this may be one of the proteins you can afford from organic sources.

- ✓ **Fish:** Fresh, wild-caught fish is a good source of protein, B-vitamins, selenium and omega-3 fats.

- ✓ **Lean meats:** When choosing beef, pork or lamb, try to buy from local farmers who raise grass-fed, antibiotic-free livestock. Doing so means you're most likely getting the highest nutrient value.

  Don't beat yourself up if the meat you buy isn't always grass-fed and organic. Not everyone can always afford to purchase this type of meat, or access it. Buy this meat when you can, but always make sure the meat you purchase is not processed and is good quality.

- ✓ **Poultry:** Don't get stuck in a boring chicken rut — turkey, duck, spatchcock, goose and quail are all delicious options too.

- ✓ **Dairy:** Milk, cottage cheese, ricotta cheese, feta cheese and plain Greek yoghurt can be decent sources of protein. Carbs are in dairy products due to the *lactose* (the sugar component of milk), but if you cut your hidden sugars from processed foods, the small amount that you get naturally occurring in dairy doesn't need to be excluded. Cheese can be high in fat, which is good in moderation, but just keep in mind that an excess of any macronutrient — protein, fat or carb — will lead to excess body fat. You can also experiment with other, more exotic, dairy proteins, like goat's milk or *kefir* (a fermented milk drink made with kefir grains) if you're feeling adventurous. One strong bonus to dairy products is the high calcium content.

Getting protein from plants

Plant protein can be an excellent source of protein. If you're eating a variety of plant proteins, you can easily attain all of the essential amino acids you need for optimal health and proper metabolism. Grains, seeds and nuts, soy, beans and legumes (such as lentils, chickpeas, black beans and kidney beans) are excellent sources of plant protein.

In the past, health experts advised that 'food combining for vegetarians' (combining specific types of plant protein in the same meal) was required to nutritionally get a complete protein like that found in animal proteins. However, most nutritionists today agree that if you have a diet with variety, the food groups you eat throughout the day will create a full set of amino acids for optimal health.

One big bonus to plant protein is that it's an excellent source of fibre and phytonutrients that you can't get from animal proteins. Keep in mind that 25 to 30 grams of fibre is the best amount for optimal digestive health.

If you're feeling acidic (such as experiencing heartburn, bad breath and joint pains), try adding some plant proteins to your diet. Plant proteins are generally more alkaline than animal proteins. In addition to being more alkalising, plant proteins may be easier to assimilate for people with digestive issues.

Soybeans (and edamame, which is just a soybean picked before it's ripe), soy milk, tofu and powdered soy protein are on the list for vegetable proteins, and can be consumed occasionally. Tempeh and miso are called *fermented* soy foods and some nutritionists believe these are the best forms of soy foods to consume. Soy may lower cholesterol and triglycerides, and some evidence exists that the *isoflavones* in soy can help prevent breast cancer.

Only choose soy-based products that are not genetically modified — the labels on all soy-based products sold in Australia and New Zealand should indicate whether they're GMO-free or organic.

If you have a thyroid issue, soy becomes the subject of considerable debate and ongoing research. Unfermented soy, organic or not, includes substances that block the synthesis of thyroid hormones and interfere with iodine metabolism, which can disrupt your thyroid function. When a yellow flag of caution has been raised in the area of nutritional research, we recommend avoiding the food in question!

Consuming carbohydrates

Carbohydrates are the body's primary fuel source. You need carbohydrates in your diet to provide energy to each cell, to feed your brain, and to fuel your muscles and organs. If you don't eat enough carbohydrates, your body will break down muscle tissue to make some!

Despite their importance, carbs have become the big bad wolf in the world of weight loss and health consciousness. Some of this thinking is justified because all carbs are definitely not created equal, but categorising carbohydrates as purely good or purely bad is inaccurate. The physiological response that you get from eating carbohydrates depends on the type, the amount, what else you eat with them and the current state of your body's chemistry — carbs are definitely not black or white!

Dietary carbohydrates are found in these foods:

- ✔ Grain products like pastas, breads and cereals
- ✔ Some milk products like yoghurt and milk; other dairy foods like cheese and cottage cheese are low in carbohydrates
- ✔ Sugars like table sugar, syrup, sweetened beverages, honey and sweets
- ✔ Vegetables, fruits and legumes

That's right, vegetables are carbohydrate sources. We counsel hundreds of people every year, and many of them are surprised to hear that. Generally, when people tell us they've 'cut out carbs', they usually mean they've stopped eating wheat and sugar. That's fine — you don't have to eat wheat or sugar to be healthy. But if you really cut out all carbohydrates, you'd soon be in metabolic trouble and very tired.

Sources of excellent complex carbs (or logs rather than twigs; refer to Chapter 1) are small portions of sweet potatoes, brown rice, basmati rice, most vegetables, wholegrain or seed crackers, brown rice crackers, quinoa and legumes.

A carb is not just a carb — you also need to consider its overall content of nutrients, fibre and kilojoules. You should aim for eating mostly vegetables (and some low-sugar fruit) because they're loaded with vitamins, minerals and fibre, and are generally very low in kilojoules. Carbohydrates from processed grains and sugary foods are generally high in kilojoules and low in fibre and nutrients. Carbs from processed grains and sugary foods without fibre and nutrients are 'dead foods'. If you want to live the good life, eat live food, not dead food.

Choosing the right fats

In the past, dietary fat was criticised as the primary contributor to obesity and heart disease. As nutrition science progressed, it became clear that dietary fat is a very important component of nutrition. We recommend you eliminate fat phobia. Your body uses fats to produce hormones, transmit nerve impulses, regulate the immune system and create cell membranes. Fat provides taste to foods and helps you feel full, and will keep your sugar cravings at bay. Fat takes a long time to digest, so it slows the release of sugar into the bloodstream.

Fat is an efficient source of food energy; each gram of dietary fat provides approximately 37 kilojoules (9 calories) of energy for the body, compared with about 16 kilojoules (4 calories) per gram from carbohydrate or protein.

Vitamins A, D, E and K are fat-soluble, meaning they can only be digested, absorbed and transported in conjunction with fats. This means those who eat no-fat or low-fat diets miss out on the immune-enhancing qualities of vitamins A, D, E and K.

If you're constantly getting colds and flus and are on a no-fat or low-fat diet, you may not be absorbing your immune system's cold-fighting vitamins. Vitamin A is an amazing nutrient for your immune system and for the health of your skin!

Avoiding bad fats

Different types of dietary fat have different effects on the body. Two types of potentially harmful dietary fat are

- **Saturated fat:** This type of fat comes mainly from animal sources of food. Too much saturated fats from animals that are fed an inflammatory diet (including GMO grains like soy and corn instead of grass and perpetual antibiotics) can raise your inflammatory markers, which increases your risk of cardiovascular disease, dementia and other health problems.

- **Trans fat:** Trans fats are a very big concern for optimal health. They're created when unsaturated fats (like oils) are heated too much, such as when food is deep-fried. Trans fats are also intentionally added to processed food by a process called *hydrogenation.* This process creates artificial fats that don't spoil as fast as naturally occurring oils, but these Frankenstein fats are toxic to the body. The Harvard School of Public Health found even 4 grams of trans fat (the amount in a doughnut) can interfere with ovulation.

  Some of the other health problems associated with trans-fat consumption are increased inflammation, increased cholesterol and triglyceride levels, disruption of the metabolism of essential fats, increased risk of diabetes and abdominal obesity linked with polycystic ovary syndrome (PCOS).

Unfortunately, food manufacturers in Australia and New Zealand don't have to list the trans-fat content of foods on their labels (although some do). If trans fats aren't listed on the label, still look out for the words *partially hydrogenated oils.* The top food offenders that may contain trans fats or partially hydrogenated oils are margarine, crackers, pies, pasties, cakes, fried foods, microwave popcorn, potato chips, biscuits and processed baked goods.

Here are some tips for minimising trans fats in your diet:

- ✔ Avoid eating fried foods and commercially baked goods.
- ✔ Don't eat foods with 'hydrogenated' in the ingredients.
- ✔ Try not to overheat any oil that you cook with.

Seeking out good fats

Not all dietary fat is harmful! You want to consume adequate amounts of healthy fats in your diet. Here are some suggestions for foods high in healthy, unsaturated fats:

- ✔ Avocado
- ✔ Fatty fish (salmon, tuna, mackerel, anchovy)
- ✔ Nuts
- ✔ Cold-pressed or first-pressed olive oil, coconut oil, flaxseed oil, sesame oil, and nut oils like walnut oil, macadamia oil and pecan oil
- ✔ Canola oil, borage oil, grapeseed oil (these are okay but keep in mind exposure to light, air or heat can cause them to *oxidise* — which means the good qualities of these oils are turned into free radicals in the body)
- ✔ Butter and ghee (in moderation)

Of particular importance are types of unsaturated fats called *omega-3* fatty acids, found primarily in fish, nuts and some oils. These have a number of heart-healthy effects, including reducing triglyceride levels, raising HDL ('good') cholesterol, 'thinning' the blood, reducing levels of homocysteine, and lowering blood pressure.

Two essential omega-3 fatty acids are found primarily in fish: *EPA (eicosapentaenoic acid)* and *DHA (docosahexaenoic acid)*. Research shows that EPA and DHA serve as powerful natural anti-inflammatory agents, lessen the effects of depression and protect the cardiovascular system. These fats are particularly important to the function of the brain and nervous system.

Technically, the body can manufacture both EPA and DHA from another essential fatty acid — *alpha-linolenic acid* (ALA), found in flaxseed oil, canola oil, soy oil and walnut oil. However, this conversion is very inefficient (less than 10 per cent), so it's virtually impossible to convert enough ALA into adequate amounts of essential fats. Fish oil (or krill oil, if you're not allergic to shellfish) supplementation seems to be the best option (see the later section 'Fish oil for essential fats' for details on supplements).

Drinking water: A vital key to craving control

The human body is mostly water. Without it, people would have no cells, no nerve impulses and no metabolic processes. Even a small amount of dehydration (2 to 3 per cent) can result in fatigue, low blood pressure, elevated heart rate, headaches, dry skin, constipation and decreased mental function.

The part of your brain that controls the thirst sensation is called the *hypothalamus*. Guess what else the hypothalamus controls? Hunger! When you're dehydrated, the hypothalamus kicks in and triggers thirst. This can also trigger food cravings, as you've probably experienced.

Drinking enough water is one of the easiest ways to keep cravings in check. Doing so also cuts down on your desire for other, less-healthy beverages. Downing a room-temperature glass of water is one of the first things you should do when a sugar craving strikes (see Chapter 9).

Healthy eating at a glance

What you eat is the biggest determinant of your health, so make smart, healthy choices. Your body deserves it! Here are the basics of a healthy, sugar-free eating plan:

1. Eat nutrient-rich foods every three to four hours:

    ✓ Healthy fats — fish oil, nuts, olive oil

    ✓ Healthy protein — whey, wild-caught fish, eggs and meat from pasture-fed animals, non-GMO soy

    ✓ Plenty of plants (low-sugar carbohydrates) — dark and brightly coloured vegetables

    ✓ Legumes and whole grains — these are complex carbs (logs) and should be consumed with some portion control (not more than one cup in a meal)

    ✓ Fruit — enjoy two pieces of fruit per day in their whole form, not juiced

2. Minimise consumption of highly processed foods.

3. At every meal, eat a *protein* and a *plant.* Don't eat too much at one time.

4. Eat breakfast every day.

5. Drink at least 1.5 to 2 litres of water throughout the day.

6. Don't eat too much food at night — eat to fuel what you plan to do for the next four hours. In particular, if you're trying to lose weight, keep complex carbs such as legumes and grains for daytime consumption. They're still carbs and all carbs, simple or complex, break down into sugar.

Don't confuse thirst for hunger! The current recommendation for water intake is approximately 1.5 to 2 litres (six to eight glasses) per day. Try this — pour water into two 1-litre jugs and see how much of it you drink on an average day. (See the later section 'Drinking clean water' for info on the pros and cons of filtered water.)

Eating Natural Foods

Your body is designed to run on natural foods like vegetables, meat, eggs, fruit, fish, nuts and seeds. When you start to stray from that nutritional foundation by eating lots of processed foods, you lose vital nutrients and consume large amounts of artificial chemicals. To make fast or packaged foods, companies add chemicals like artificial flavouring, chemical colouring, preservatives, emulsifiers, hydrogenated oils, high-fructose corn syrup and other cheap sweeteners to extend shelf life and add 'taste'. Sticking with natural foods instead of processed foods delivers more nutrition and less sugar, preservatives, artificial flavours and colours, and other chemicals.

In this section, we explain the difference between organic and conventional produce and fill you in on the important differences between food that comes from pasture-fed, antibiotic-free animals and food from industrial feedlot operations.

Picking produce

Just 60 or 70 years ago, farmers used crop rotation and manure to keep their soil healthy. Today, the industrial agriculture business uses chemical fertilisers in the ground and covers genetically modified (or GM) plants with pesticides and herbicides. After the food is harvested, the companies treat the produce with additional chemicals to delay ripening and prevent spoilage while the food is shipped halfway across the world! The nutrition content of this produce is severely compromised. Buying organic produce from local farmers (or growing your own!) ensures that you get the freshest, most nutritious food available, without all the added chemicals. You also get produce that's picked at its peak ripeness, making it more appealing to eat!

At the time of writing, the only genetically modified food crops produced in Australia are canola and cotton. No fresh fruit, vegetables or meat sold in New Zealand is genetically modified. However, many GM foods are being imported or used as ingredients in packaged or processed foods in both countries.

Not everyone can afford organic so don't stress if you can't. Flip to Chapter 6 for advice on organic versus conventional produce. Eating whole foods like vegetables, fruits and nuts is important for vitamins, minerals, fibre and phytonutrients, whether they're organic or not!

You should seek out vegetables that aren't genetically modified — *Non-GMO* is the term to look for. Because no-one knows the long-term health consequences of engineered food, GMO food has been banned in all of Europe. Our take on foods that we're not 100 per cent sure on the health implications for is to consider this a yellow flag. Exercise caution and avoid these foods — after all, plenty of other food choices are available that you can be sure are 100 per cent healthy and safe. ***Note:*** If a food product contains ingredients that have been genetically modified, this must be included on the product's label in Australia and New Zealand.

Buying meat, dairy, eggs and fish

Animals in commercial feedlot facilities are fed unnatural foods loaded with antibiotics so that the animals fatten quicker and can survive the diseases that crowded, infected living conditions produce. Eating these types of animal products may increase inflammation in your body and raises your risk of heart disease and cancer.

Here are some tips for choosing healthier animal products:

- ✔ **Fish and seafood:** Wild-caught seafood is a great source of protein and essential fats. Generally speaking, Australian and New Zealand fish is safe to eat and Food Standards Australia New Zealand (FSANZ) regularly monitor mercury levels. Sadly, some oceans have become contaminated with mercury, polychlorinated biphenyls (PCBs) and other poisons. Fish farming also has its potential problems, because not all countries adhere to the same standards and some may use undesirable antibiotics and pesticides. The Australian Marine Conservation Society offers a downloadable sustainable seafood guide covering more than 100 seafood species to help you decide which fish is the healthiest for you — access the guide at sustainableseafood.com.au.

If you love the convenience of canned tuna and salmon but are rightly concerned about the mercury levels, FSANZ advises that people, including pregnant women, can safely eat two to three serves per week of any type of tuna or salmon — canned or fresh. FSANZ does advise it's better to eat smaller species of fish rather than the large species at the top of the food chain. (This is also why canned tuna usually has lower levels of mercury than other tuna — the tuna caught for canning is usually a smaller species and less than one year old.) For more information go to www.foodauthority.nsw.gov.au and search for 'canned tuna'.

✔ **Meat and dairy:** Organic, free-range livestock (and the dairy foods from them) have a better nutrition profile — more healthy fats and nutrients and potentially less inflammatory chemicals — than food from commercial feedlot animals, so try to buy your food from local organic or pasture-fed farms.

Organic certification can be very expensive in Australia and New Zealand, so don't be fooled into thinking that pasture-fed isn't as good as organic. Certified Organic is the audited guarantee that the product is free-range and grass-fed. However, some locally grown uncertified livestock is pasture-fed and free-range — the farmers just may not have been able to afford the organic certification and may be spending money on sustainable farming instead. Husbandry claims should be carefully checked on a local level.

About 70 per cent of Australian and New Zealand beef and lamb is pasture-fed, unlike the United States, where grain-fed is a much bigger issue. Grain-fed animals are often treated with antibiotics, kept in feedlots, and fed corn and soy grains. These grains are often genetically modified and are used to fatten up the animals before they die. Sadly, farmers often put pasture-fed animals on grain 5 to 120 days before slaughter to 'plump' them up. Try to buy meat you know is 100 per cent pasture-fed — this is usually referred to as 'grass-fed and finished'.

✔ **Poultry and eggs:** Aim to buy poultry raised without antibiotics in their feed. Whenever possible, choose eggs from pasture-fed chickens, which have less cholesterol and more vitamins and omega-3s (and the living conditions for chickens in industrial operations are atrocious).

Drinking clean water

Filtered water and distilled water is the subject of great discussion among health-care professionals. Our recommendation is to drink the majority of your water either from filtered or distilled water. Water filters remove some of the large contaminants and bacteria, and distilling water can eliminate mercury, lead, pesticides, pharmaceutical residue, PCBs, livestock runoff and other hazards that seep into the groundwater. Feel confident that you can get your minerals and alkalinity from nutrient-dense food.

Water bottle companies often clean water using a purification system with carbon filtration, ozonation and reverse osmosis. If you're purchasing bottled water, only consider glass bottles. Plastic water bottles can leach bisphenol A (BPA), an endocrine disruptor that may lead to negative health effects, into your 'clean' water!

Managing Kilojoules and Portion Control

In nutrition, a *kilojoule* is the measure of the amount of energy contained in a food. In Australia and New Zealand, the metric (kilojoule) system is used; however, people commonly still use 'calories' when referring to the energy content of foods. The energy content is required to be declared on most packaged foods in either kilojoules or both kilojoules and calories.

Your body breaks down foods (burns kilojoules) to provide energy to move, think and keep all the metabolic processes going. The three macronutrients (protein, fat and carbohydrate) have kilojoules. Protein and carbohydrates contain approximately 17 kilojoules (kJ) or 4 calories (Cal) per gram. Fat has 37 kilojoules (9 Cal) and alcohol has 29 kJ (7 Cal) per gram.

In this section, we explore the quality of kilojoules, find out how many kilojoules you need, and look at what size your portions should be.

Realising that a kilojoule isn't just a kilojoule

One of the common nutrition mantras that continues to spew from pop medical publications is that the only thing that determines weight loss or weight gain is kilojoules in versus kilojoules out. This is just not true — what happens to the kilojoules you eat is highly dependent on what kind of kilojoules they are and on the physiological state of the eater.

Let's take two subjects as examples: Woman A splits up 4,800 kilojoules of vegetables and lean protein into five meals every day. Woman B doesn't eat during the day and then gobbles 4,800 kilojoules' worth of doughnuts every night before bed. These two women will have very different bodies and health profiles, even though they both eat the same number of kilojoules every day. A kilojoule is *not* just a kilojoule!

To stay healthy and lean, be sure to take in most of your kilojoules from high-nutrient foods, not *empty kilojoules* (kilojoules without nutrition value).

Determining how many kilojoules you need

If you eat more kilojoules than you need, your body stores the excess as fat. Sugar is a particularly troublesome source of kilojoules because it's often very low in nutrients, robs you of good nutrients and triggers cravings for even more.

When you regularly eat more energy than your body needs, the excess is stored inside fat cells. Just 1 kilogram of body fat contains the equivalent of 37,000 kJ. To lose 1 kilogram of body fat in a week, you would need to burn an additional 37,000 kJ, or around 5,000 kJ a day!

Individual kilojoule requirements vary greatly depending on personal metabolism and activity levels, but you can get a decent ballpark number from combining your Basal Metabolic Rate (BMR) with the Harris-Benedict formula. Here's how it works:

✔ **BMR:** First calculate your BMR with the following:

Women = 655 + (9.6 × weight in kilograms) + (1.8 × height in centimetres) − (4.7 × age in years)

Men = 66 + (13.7 × weight in kilograms) + (5 × height in centimetres) − (6.8 × age in years)

✔ **The Harris-Benedict formula:** You then use your BMR to determine your daily calorie needs to maintain your current weight, as follows:

- If your lifestyle is sedentary (with little or no exercise), multiply your BMR by 1.2.

- If you're lightly active (you participate in light exercise or sports one to 3 days per week), multiply your BMR by 1.375.

- If you're moderately active (you participate in moderate exercise or sports three to five days per week), multiply your BMR by 1.55.

- If you're very active (you participate in hard exercise or sports six to seven days per week), multiply your BMR by 1.725.

- If you're extra active (you participate in very hard exercise or sports and have a physical job, or are training twice a day), multiply your BMR by 1.9.

If you do not like maths, go to www.healthyweightforum.org/eng/calculators/calories-required to easily find out your total kilojoules needs. But remember — we believe that once you begin this journey of low sugar and whole foods, you will stop counting calories and start enjoying the new you.

A balanced diet: Finding the right ratios

For years, Australians and New Zealanders have been duped into believing that a grain-based, low-fat diet is the best way to combat obesity. As the consistent and appalling rise in obesity and diabetes continues, it's clear that a new set of nutrition guidelines is in order.

In 2013, Australia's National Health and Medical Research Council (NHMRC) released the *Australian Guide to Healthy Eating*, which is a considerable improvement from the old-school food pyramids of the past. The new guide recommends three to seven servings of grains per day. This may still seem overly generous, but the serving sizes are often small compared to the actual amount eaten. For example, two slices of bread is equal to two serves. For a copy of the guide, go to health.gov.au and search for 'Australian Guide to Healthy Eating'. ***Note:*** Unfortunately, the guidelines don't feature quality fats.

The last update to the New Zealand Food and Nutrition Guidelines was in 2003, so we recommend following the more up-to-date Australian guidelines.

The MyPlate recommendations (www.chooseMyplate.gov, © U.S. Department of Agriculture), shown in Figure 5-1, advise that half your plate should be filled with vegetables and fruits, one quarter with protein, and one quarter with grains, along with a serving of dairy. The new guidelines are reasonable but still not ideal due to the exclusion of quality fats.

'Guidelines' are just that — guidelines. They don't take into account a person's health history or nutritional goals (like reducing sugar).

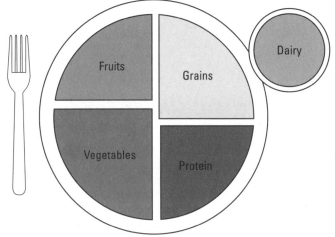

Figure 5-1: MyPlate food guidelines.

Illustration by Wiley, Composition Services Graphics

By combining current available research and many years of experience in nutrition counselling, we have determined that *most individuals* with average kilojoule expenditure — which means somewhere between completely sedentary and moderately active — function best with approximately equal ratios of kilojoules from protein, fat and carbohydrate in the diet, creating the 30/30/40 plate shown in Figure 5-2. *Note:* We emphasis 'most individuals' because everyone's body metabolism is different and some people will function on very different ratios.

If you can eat 30 per cent of your kilojoules from protein, 30 per cent from healthy fats and 40 per cent from carbohydrates (mostly vegetables), you can stay lean, healthy and craving-free! This type of insulin-controlled eating is not just for those with diabetes — it's for anyone who would like mental clarity, balanced hormones, optimal weight, vitality and consistent energy levels!

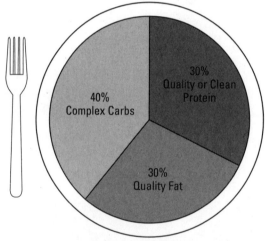

Figure 5-2:
The 30/30/40 plate.

Illustration by Wiley, Composition Services Graphics

Portion distortion: Understanding how much is too much

Increased kilojoule consumption is one of the three primary causes of obesity in Australia and New Zealand (along with increased sugar consumption and lack of physical activity). Portions and kilojoule content have risen consistently over the decades, and Aussies and Kiwis have the waistlines to prove it!

Here are some comparisons of portion sizes in the 1980s versus today:

Portions and Kilojoules in the 1980s	Portions and Kilojoules Today
One 250-millilitre coffee with milk and sugar: 377 kilojoules	Frappuccino: 500 millilitres, 1,647 kilojoules
Blueberry muffin: 40 grams, 879 kilojoules	Blueberry muffin:140 grams, 2,092 kilojoules
Chicken stir-fry: 2 cups, 1,820 kilojoules	Chicken stir-fry: 4 cups, 3,556 kilojoules
Raisin toast: 2 slices regular size, 806 kilojoules	Raisin toast: 2 slices thick, 1,962 kilojoules

Note: Sizes and measures may vary slightly.

To become accustomed to what a normal serving size is, put out your usual portion of food, measure it, and then compare your serving size to what's on the nutrition label. You may be surprised (or maybe horrified?) to find that your 'normal' portion of pasta or breakfast cereal is actually three or four servings!

Manufacturers often try to disguise the amount of sugar in their products by using small serving sizes on their labels, so finding your portion size is the same size as what's on the label may be unusual.

To become more skilled at eyeballing portions, refer to your hand for appropriate sizes; you may not always have a scale but you will always have your hand. Use the following as a guide:

- ✔ Your fist = a serving of starch like pasta, potatoes or rice
- ✔ Your fist = a serving of fruit
- ✔ Palm of your hand = a serving of grainy, dark bread
- ✔ Palm of your hand = a serving of meat or fish
- ✔ Inside your fist = a serving of nuts (pop the nuts in your hand and close it — what falls out was not meant to be eaten)
- ✔ Half your thumb (knuckle to tip) = 1 teaspoon

We're not asking you to go to the effort of measuring your food for the long term. However, try it for one week — this will be long enough for you to get a sense of what a portion size truly looks like. Then we recommend getting rid of the scales. Food is meant to be enjoyed and not to be obsessed over, dissected and tightly measured. Once you have transitioned to a low-sugar way of life, the process becomes a habit, and you begin to trust that you can eat whole, unpackaged foods, real food, without having to worry about your weight.

Adding Supplements for Health and Help

Fortifying your diet with the right nutrition supplements can help fend off sugar cravings and add a much-needed boost to your health and vitality. Proper supplementation is an important component of long-term health and wellness because it's difficult to obtain all the vitamins, minerals, essential fats and phytonutrients that you need to defend against the onslaught of dangerous chemicals found in the food supply and the environment.

These days your body simply has more to deal with — more stress, more chemicals, more radiation and more pollutants. To stay healthy, you need serious help, including stress management, smart choices in food, and extra nutrition support.

In addition to choosing nutritious, chemical-free foods (see the earlier section 'Eating Natural Foods' for details), you may want to consider the nutrition supplements explained in the next few sections.

These nutrition supplements may not be appropriate for every individual. Some nutrients can cause problems in people with certain medical conditions or can interact with particular medications. You should always consult a qualified practitioner for advice concerning your individual requirements.

Multivitamin/mineral supplement with B-complex

Farming practices and chemical fertilisers have depleted the mineral content of the soil in Australia and New Zealand. Organic farming has begun a positive turnaround, but it will take decades for the soil to recover. To ensure that your body has the necessary amounts of the missing minerals — nutrients like chromium, selenium, magnesium and copper that are no longer in the soil — you can use a basic multivitamin/mineral supplement for nutritional insurance. Remember that deficiencies in nutrients can trigger cravings!

The B-vitamins are critical for energy production, dopamine and serotonin production, and brain function. B-vitamins have been shown to lower the risk of diabetes and to decrease the incidence of migraines. If your multivitamin/mineral supplement doesn't contain B-vitamins, you can take an additional B-complex separately.

Recommended brands of quality multivitamin/mineral supplements are available at www.ahealthyview.com.au.

Vitamin C, an immune booster

Infections and stress eat up vitamin C. Supplemental vitamin C boosts your immunity by improving components of the immune system that have cool-sounding names like *natural killer cells* and *lymphocytes*. Vitamin C helps maintain the integrity of cells and helps protect them against oxidative damage (similar to rusting on the inside). Vitamin C is also important for iron absorption, wound healing and maintaining the strength of blood capillaries, and is very important to collagen synthesis — in other words, preventing wrinkles!

An interesting fact: Humans are one of the few mammals that can't make their own vitamin C. The others are apes, guinea pigs and fruit bats.

If you're new to vitamin C supplements, use a dose of up to 1,000 milligrams. Large doses of vitamin C can cause diarrhoea if you're unaccustomed to it.

Fish oil for essential fats

Fish oil is one of the only concentrated forms of essential fats. Essential omega-3 fats are powerful, natural, anti-inflammatory agents, and they help repair nerve and brain cells, regulate the immune system and even improve mood.

The typical dosage is 1 to 3 grams of distilled fish oil daily. Buy fish oil capsules that have been molecularly distilled to remove toxins like mercury, pesticides and PCBs. You can find a current list of recommended brands at www.ahealthyview.com.au.

If you experience stomach upset or fishy burps, try an enteric-coated fish oil capsule. Both fish oil and krill oil supplements supply omega-3 fatty acids, DHA and EPA. Krill comes from small crustaceans, not fatty fish, and often contains more EPA.

Fish oil has a mild blood-thinning effect. If you use prescription blood thinners like Warfarin or Plavix, consult a knowledgeable nutritionist or health-care professional before supplementing with fish oil.

Whey protein to help stabilise blood sugar

Powdered whey protein can be an additional source of protein. Our preference would always be real food first but a good quality, 'clean' protein powder can be quick, filling and nutritious.

Choose a *whey protein concentrate* supplement that is 'clean'. We define a clean whey protein powder as one that has **no**

- ✔ Antibiotics
- ✔ Chemical additives
- ✔ Colour additives
- ✔ Fructose
- ✔ Genetically modified ingredients
- ✔ Gluten
- ✔ High-fructose corn syrup
- ✔ Hydrolysed proteins
- ✔ MSG
- ✔ Pesticides
- ✔ Preservatives
- ✔ Soy
- ✔ Sucralose
- ✔ Sugar added
- ✔ Sugar alcohols

Eating protein slows down the insulin response when you eat (which is good) and helps maintain blood sugar levels after you eat. Eating enough protein is one of the primary ways to keep the carb cravings away and mood and energy slumps at bay.

Whey protein contains *immunoglobulins*, which boost the performance of your immune system. Whey protein also has a high concentration of *glutamine*, an amino acid that's a vital component of the immune system.

Clients often tell us that one of their challenges is getting a protein source every time they eat. Whey protein is a quick and easy way to get your protein — add a scoop to your porridge, put it in your smoothie, or whip up a protein shake for a snack. Michele's clients often like to make a quick berry smoothie with protein powder for their afternoon tea to stomp out the afternoon cravings.

Because the whey powder you choose should have no artificial sweeteners, flavour should come from sources that add functional benefits — cinnamon or pure vanilla are good examples. Consult a practitioner if you're not sure and be wary of inexpensive brands coming from overseas that 'guarantee weight loss and massive muscle'. You can find a list of recommended brands at www.ahealthyview.com.au.

Probiotics: The good bacteria

Humans have lots of different types of bacteria (sometimes referred to as *intestinal flora*) in the digestive tract, and these bacteria are an integral part of both the digestive and immune systems. The intestinal flora also keeps other insidious things from colonising in the gut.

These beneficial bacteria are often killed off by antibiotics, poor diet, illness or stress. This is a major problem because a lack of beneficial bacteria in the gut can cause a host of problems with both digestion and immunity.

Taking a probiotic supplement is an easy way to help maintain the proper levels of favourable bacteria in your body. These are small capsules containing billions of helpful organisms to improve lactose intolerance, bloating, flatulence and constipation, and improve symptoms of inflammatory gastrointestinal conditions (IBS, colitis, Crohn's), erase eczema, reduce allergies, improve your immune system response and clear up ulcers from *Helicobacter pylori* bacteria.

Typical probiotic capsules contain between 1 and 3 billion active organisms. For general health and immune system support, a daily dose of 1 to 5 billion organisms is generally sufficient. If you're combating a yeast infection, replenishing the gut after a course of antibiotics or using probiotics for another therapeutic function, you may have to temporarily use a larger dose of 10 to 30 billion organisms per day. Consult a knowledgeable health-care professional for advice.

Some probiotic supplements contain only two or three strains of bacteria. A more effective choice is a brand that contains many different strains.

Green drinks for extra vegetables

One of the difficulties reported to us on a regular basis is getting enough vegetables in the diet. A powdered green drink is an alternative way to put some more *phytonutrients* (plant nutrients) into your daily diet. If you're finding it difficult to fit in vegetables at every meal, think about starting your day with Thr1ve Performa Greens.

Dozens of companies sell vegetable and fruit powder. Be sure to choose a 'clean' one without added sugars, fillers or artificial sweeteners! A good green drink should include lots of different plants, such as spirulina, chlorella, wheatgrass, flaxseed, alfalfa, barley, broccoli, dandelion and spinach.

If you like to juice vegetables yourself, be sure to vary your concoctions from day to day so that you get a wide variety of nutrients in your diet. Personally, we prefer to eat our vegetables whole, but the occasional juice is a very nice treat. The general rule is, the more colour, the greater the antioxidant value. If you choose to juice, use a quality juicer to ensure you're keeping the nutrients and as much fibre as possible. See www.ahealthyview.com.au for what to look for in a juicer.

Magnesium for relaxed muscles and strong bones

Nutritionally we call magnesium 'the great calmer'. Low levels of magnesium can make muscles shorten and spasm, causing achiness or muscle cramps. Magnesium relaxes muscles, improves sleep and relieves tension.

According to a study published in *Diabetes Care,* magnesium deficiency can contribute to obesity and insulin resistance. High magnesium intake gives you a 30 per cent less chance of developing metabolic syndrome too!

Magnesium helps keep your blood pressure normal and your heart rhythm steady. It's also a crucial mineral in the formation of bone tissue — anyone using a calcium supplement for osteoporosis should be sure that the supplement also contains magnesium (along with vitamin D, boron and vitamin K2).

Studies show that overweight adults over age 40 who consumed less than 50 per cent of the recommended amount of magnesium were twice as likely to have increased systemic inflammation, which contributes to major health problems such as heart disease, diabetes and cancer.

Magnesium is also involved in the production of the three 'happiness' neurotransmitters: serotonin, dopamine and norepinephrine.

The recommended dosage of supplemental magnesium is 200 to 400 milligrams per day. Look for magnesium gluconate, magnesium aspartate (or another amino acid chelate), or magnesium citrate.

Two other sources of magnesium are Rooibos tea and Epsom salt baths. So draw yourself a bath, dissolve half a cup of salts in it, and sip some Rooibos tea by candle light — and be prepared for a calming night's sleep.

Chapter 6

Stocking a Low-Sugar Kitchen

. . . .

In This Chapter

▶ Creating a healthy, low-sugar kitchen

▶ Keeping good sources of protein and the right carbs on hand

▶ Making a grocery list and reading nutrition labels

▶ Eating healthier foods on a budget

. . . .

*T*hose who plan, plan to succeed. If you don't believe that statement, think back to a time when you succeeded in life. Now ask yourself — did it take some type of planning? Your kitchen is the control centre of your nutrition universe; it's where you plan, store and create the foods that make or break your healthy way of life (notice that we didn't write make or break your *diet*). If you don't stock your refrigerator and pantry with nutritious food from which to feed yourself and your family, you leave yourself and your loved ones at the mercy of chemical-laden fast foods and perilous takeaway meals. Planning and purposeful eating are the cornerstones of beating sugar addiction, and your kitchen needs to be an organised nutrition sanctuary for you to maintain long-term success. Stock it well with delicious and nutritious foods so you don't miss your old pantry.

This chapter is full of information to help you perform a total kitchen makeover. You'll find suggestions for how to stay organised and prepared, and for the kinds of healthy foods you should stock in your refrigerator, pantry and freezer. We suggest what to buy at the grocery store and supermarket, and show you how to decipher the nutrition facts labels. You'll also discover how to identify some of the hidden sources of sugars in many common foods, and find out when spending a little extra on organic and local food is worth the money.

Cleaning Out the Cabinets, Fridge and Freezer

Everyone is a creature of habit, and the overloaded schedule that most people struggle with demands convenient and time-efficient meals. To successfully implement an improved eating plan, you must make sure that healthy, low-sugar foods are available in your home. If your kitchen and pantry are filled with unhealthy food, your overloaded brain will drive you there when you finally take a moment to eat something. You're most likely going to eat whatever is handy, so the first step in upgrading to a healthier kitchen is to remove the non-nutritious food and stock a supply of quality food instead. Your goal is to make eating healthy food easy for you to do on a consistent basis.

Tossing out the obvious culprits

If you don't keep junk food in your house, you won't have to worry about resisting the temptation to dive in! Get rid of these obvious sugar culprits:

- Agave nectar (high fructose!)
- Bakery items that are store bought and processed, such as muffins, cakes, pies and doughnuts
- Biscuits
- Honey
- Lollies and ice cream
- Packaged breakfast cereals
- Soft drinks and other sweetened drinks, including juice drinks, juice poppers, flavoured milk, diet soft drinks, cordial, prepackaged tea drinks and energy drinks
- Table sugar

Next, look at the labels on the jars in the pantry and fridge. Toss (actually, empty and recycle) bottles or sauces that have a first or second ingredient that's 'sugar' (or similar — refer to Chapter 3 for a complete list).

If you'd like to take things a step further or if you're dealing with blood sugar problems like diabetes, you can also remove white-flour products.

Still drawn to white-flour products, or know someone in your family who is? Think about the playdough you played with at kindergarten, or perhaps made for your kids. What is it primarily made of? White flour, water and salt. What is white bread primarily made of? The same key ingredients. Would you eat a ball of fibreless, dead playdough? Then why would you eat fibreless, low-nutrient, belly- and bowel-clogging white bread?

Uncovering less-obvious troublemakers

Sugar is prevalent in the Western food supply, and it comes in many forms, with many different names. Cutting back on how much sugar you eat isn't always easy if you're not aware of how sugars can be disguised on the list of ingredients. When you're looking at labels and deciding what to keep or discard, consult the nearby sidebar 'Other names for sugar' and Chapter 3 for many alternative names for sugar.

The first place to look when seeking out hidden sugar is in foods that are otherwise considered healthy. Though yoghurts, fruit juice, protein bars and muesli have more nutrients than empty-calorie junk food, if you look at the nutrition facts you'll find that most of them are laden with sugars. The fact that a food contains vitamins and antioxidants or is gluten-free and/or fat-free doesn't make it sugar-free!

Fruit juice and other drinks

Fruit juice contains a lot of concentrated fructose because none of the fruit pulp or fibre is present. Concentrated fructose is a direct path to obesity and diabetes, so while 100 per cent fruit juice may be high in vitamins and antioxidants, you should drink it sparingly, if at all. Eat your fruit, don't drink it.

Choice, the Australian consumer advocacy group, has found that a quarter of the juice box products sold in Australia (often known as 'poppers') contain 25 per cent or less juice. Rates are similar for products sold in New Zealand. While they may be convenient in the lunchbox, juice box products really are nothing more than a sweet drink. Juice drinks are far worse than real fruit juice because they have all the calories and fructose but none of the nutrients of natural fruit juice. Juice boxes may also be loaded with artificial colouring and preservatives.

Many flavoured milks contain as much if not more sugar than many soft drinks. Australians and New Zealanders love their flavoured milk but these drinks don't have the nutritional equivalent of unflavoured milk. They're higher in kilojoules and sugar, and often contain artificial colours and flavours.

Flavoured milks can have more sugar than a large chocolate bar or a can of soft drink. At one of Michele's recent school presentations, one of the teenagers in the audience was drinking banana-flavoured milk. It's wonderful when teenagers (or adults for that matter) can see a real life, timely example of hidden sugars. This teenager came up in front of his peers and said that he was embarrassed to admit he had just drunk 13 teaspoons of sugar in five minutes while gulping his morning milk. He also commented that he might not have the caramel-flavoured milk for lunch that day!

Diet drinks

Even though a diet soda shows zero calories and zero sugar on the label, you should stay away from these dangerous beverages. Chemical sweeteners are proven health hazards and appetite stimulants (refer to Chapter 3), artificial caramel colouring is a carcinogen, and the phosphoric acid in soft drinks leaches calcium out of your bones. Whether sweetened or unsweetened, soft drinks don't have a single redeeming quality, so stay away!

If you love the fizziness of soft drinks, try mineral water flavoured with mint or a slice of lemon or lime instead.

As you work to wean yourself off sugar, consider using *stevia powder* as a low-calorie sweetener instead of NutraSweet, saccharin or any other chemical concoction. But try to only use it as you transition to low sugar; the long-term effects of stevia aren't known yet and, more importantly in our experience, sweet tastes create sweet cravings and the vicious cycle continues. If you're using stevia in the short term, be sure to read the label to confirm that the brand of stevia you buy has no added sugars or artificial sweeteners, and isn't bleached.

Other names for sugar

When you're looking at labels and deciding what to keep or discard, be on the lookout for these common names for sugar:

- Barley malt
- Dehydrated cane juice
- Dextrose
- Evaporated cane juice
- Fructose
- Fruit juice concentrate
- Maltodextrin
- Molasses
- Sucrose

You can find a more complete list of alternative names for sugar in Chapter 3.

Skipping low-fat options

Australia and New Zealand went through a huge fat-free food craze in the 1990s. Because fat-free food was in demand, food manufacturers added sugar and other flavourings to make up for the taste of the missing fat. At the time, most people didn't think about calories or sugar content; they were only focused on cutting back on the number of fat grams they ate. As a result, the amount of sugar consumed has skyrocketed, obesity rates have doubled, and diabetes has become an epidemic.

Dietary fat is important for a host of vital functions in your body (refer to Chapter 5), including producing hormones, conducting nerve impulses, regulating your immune system, absorbing certain vitamins and building cell membranes. Dietary fat has the important job of slowing down the breakdown of carbohydrates in your digestive system, so you get a smaller insulin response when you eat fat with your food. Low-fat, high-carb eating increases the amount of insulin that your body produces, leading to obesity and insulin resistance. Perhaps you're struggling to believe such a significant shift in the thinking on weight loss and optimal health, but trust us — some dietary fat is good for you.

Fat has more calories per gram than carbohydrates or protein, so eating fat helps you feel full. As discussed in Chapter 3, eating a low-fat, high-carb diet puts you on the blood sugar roller-coaster, stimulating your appetite and activating sugar cravings.

While some nutritionists advocate saturated and unsaturated fats are fine in your diets, we recommend sticking mostly to *monounsaturated fats*. Fish oil, extra-virgin or cold-pressed olive oils and nut oils, avocados, nuts and seeds contain monounsaturated fats that minimise your exposure to inflammatory trans fats from hydrogenated oils and saturated fats from feedlot meat and dairy.

Eliminating questionable foods

When in doubt, throw it out (or donate it). All you really need to eat to be healthy each day is quality protein, a large variety of organic (if possible) vegetables, a couple of pieces of fruit, and some essential dietary fat from fish oil, nuts and extra-virgin or cold-pressed olive oil. Most of your food every day should be composed of these simple, natural items. If you're pulling your hair out trying to decipher labels and count sugar grams, stop fretting about the details and make things really simple for yourself: If it's not a protein, a plant or a healthy fat, don't eat it and don't buy it for your family. If it's processed, wrapped or boxed, read the label before you decide that you want that food to become part of you.

Inevitably, you'll find yourself out and about when you haven't planned well and you need to grab some not-so-healthy food, so don't stock that stuff in your house. If your day-to-day food is healthy and sugar-free, you won't have to take an extreme view when you're eating out at special occasions.

If you're going to get rid of a lot of extra food that you don't want in the house any more, don't waste it. In Australia, you can donate your pantry items to various charities in your state or territory — see www.givenow.com.au/ otherways/food for a list of options close to you. In New Zealand you can donate food through the Salvation Army — go to salvationarmy.org.nz/ support-us/food-banks for more information.

Creating a Sugar-Smart Kitchen

The keys to staying on track with a healthy eating system are to plan ahead and to make sure that healthy foods are available and convenient. After you use the guidelines in the previous section to remove the sugar-infused food from your pantry, refrigerator and freezer, it's time to refill them with upgraded food choices.

Making a food plan for the next few days (or the next week) is an important way to stay on track with your healthy eating system — once again, without a plan, you'll find it difficult to succeed. As Michele often says to her clients, 'A vision without a plan is just a wish, but a vision with a plan happens!' Search online for recipes using whole foods and plan out all your meals, so you can then shop and prepare foods accordingly.

Stocking up on protein

Protein and vegetables are your two best friends when it comes to staying sugar-free. Protein slows down the absorption of carbohydrates into the bloodstream and helps you feel satisfied for longer periods of time. Protein is important for myriad other functions in your body, which you can read about in Chapter 5.

A sugar-smart kitchen should have two main sources of protein handy:

- ✔ Fish, chicken, meat and eggs (wild-caught, pasture-fed and organic are ideal if possible) in the freezer and refrigerator for planned meals. Nuts and seeds are excellent to have in the pantry too.

- ✔ Powdered 'clean' whey protein (for last-minute snacks or for whenever you need a handy source of additional protein). Visit www.ahealthyview.com.au for current brand recommendations.

When you make your food plan for the next day or two (or for the week), be sure to make notes about when to move frozen meats into the refrigerator so they're thawed when it's time to cook them.

We recommend buying meats from a trusted butcher, farm or organic brand when possible. Of course, this may not be possible all the time — everyone is busy, after all, and you may be more limited with options where you live. Also, if you make finding and sourcing food difficult, your whole nutritional transformation may come undone. So just do what you can and have some sense of awareness about what you are buying to nourish yourself. The food seems to taste better when you know where it is from. See the 'Eating local: Farmers' markets' section later in this chapter for more info.

Tips for buying and cooking healthy fish

Whenever possible, you should buy fish that's wild-caught instead of farmed. Experts claim that 50 per cent of fish purchased in Australia and New Zealand comes from farming due to sustainability issues. We understand these factors but still recommend you should try to purchase what is closest to nature, for the following reasons:

✔ Farm-raised fish may contain higher amounts of pro-inflammatory omega-6 fats than wild fish due to the ingredients of the fish pellet.

✔ Farmed fish are often raised in crowded commercial tanks and are, therefore, prone to disease and parasites. Fish farmers add antibiotics and pesticides and some even vaccinate them!

✔ Farmed fish contain less beneficial omega-3 fats than wild fish, but have a much higher fat content by weight.

✔ Farmed fish may contain dangerous chemicals like polychlorinated biphenyls (PCBs) and dioxins.

✔ Some salmon are fed a pink-coloured dye to change the colour of their flesh.

✔ Fish farming can have drastic effects on wild fish — 95 per cent of wild fish will die if they contact water infested with a fish farm's sea lice.

✔ Wild salmon have an average of 20 per cent more protein than farmed salmon — they're not artificially fattened like farmed salmon.

You can reduce some of the contaminants in fish by cutting off the skin and fat before cooking. Grill fish on a rack so the fat drips off the fish, and don't use fish drippings for sauces. Don't eat fish organs or the dark patches of fish meat, because more contaminants collect there.

To reduce the consumption of mercury in fish, avoid eating large predatory fish like shark, swordfish or king mackerel. White tuna (larger fish) generally has more mercury than light tuna, although levels vary widely. Smaller fish like squid, oysters, mackerel, sardines and mussels are safer choices. The US National Resources Defence Council has an excellent card on the mercury levels of fish, available at www.nrdc.org/health/effects/mercury/walletcard.pdf. (The card also shows which types of fish are endangered or caught using environmentally destructive practices.)

For more information about environmentally responsible seafood do's and don'ts, visit www.nrdc.org/oceans/seafoodguide/default.asp or www.fish.govt.nz/en-nz/default.htm.

Finding the right carbs

Most of the carbohydrates you eat should come from vegetables. Vegetables are low in calories and sugar and high in nutrients and fibre. You can pretty much eat all the veggies you want without having to worry about calories or insulin response.

All vegetables contain some level of fructose (with beets being the highest, followed by peas and carrots) but the fructose in vegetables isn't such a worry due to their high fibre content. So a bad vegetable doesn't exist. Don't get caught up in the low-starch or high-starch vegetable debate. If you choose daily from a variety of vegetables you'll generally get a healthy mix of both. To make preparing vegetables easy, keep your refrigerator stocked with fresh, crunchy produce ready to lightly sauté, stir-fry, grill, steam or eat raw. When fresh vegetables aren't in season, you can buy frozen vegetables for quick and easy cooking or pick up a bag of prewashed organic salad mix for a mixed green salad.

We don't recommend that you use canned vegetables because they're often high in sodium and can contain contaminants like bisphenol-a (BPA).

Keep a see-through container of raw, cut vegetables in the refrigerator. For a snack or an appetiser, dip raw, crunchy vegetables in extra-virgin or cold-pressed olive oil, salsa, hummus, or a yoghurt-based dip like tzatziki.

Here are some more tips for including more vegetables into your meal planning:

- ✔ Add a side of vegetables to each of your meals and don't just steam them. Stir-fry them with garlic and chilli, grill them with sea salt and lemon rind, bake them with red onions and shallots, or crunch some raw. Make them exciting!

- ✔ Include a mixed green salad with your meal at least once per day. Make your salad exciting. Peel some lemon or lime rind, shave some fennel, chop some celery, add some crunchy sprouts and have fun with some dressings. Mustards mixed with olive oil or plain walnut or macadamia nut oils can make a boring salad quite tasty.

- ✔ Embellish your vegetables with nutrient-dense spices like chilli, garlic, lemon rind, pepper, lemon myrtle, rosemary, cumin and oregano. See www.thespicetradingcompany.com.au for an amazing array of tasty spices.

- ✔ Prepare double servings of vegetables each time you cook them so that you have leftovers in your refrigerator for quick omelette or quiche fillings.

- ✔ Shred carrots or zucchini into meatloaf, casseroles and muffins.

Store your vegetables to ensure they last for longer and retain their nutrients and taste. Store them in see-through containers in the fridge, or use some of the commercially available salad and vegetable containers. See `www.ahealthyview.com.au` for some options.

Discovering satisfying beverages

One of the difficulties reported by many sugar addicts is staying away from soft drinks (refer to the 'Diet drinks' section earlier in the chapter). To transition away from sweetened drinks, you can start incorporating mineral water flavoured with fresh citrus, or investigate the endless varieties of teas you can brew.

Avoid drinking energy drinks, bottled teas or sports drinks because they're usually loaded with sugar (or artificial sweeteners), caffeine and chemical additives.

An easy way to reduce the frequency of sugar cravings is to make sure that you stay hydrated throughout the day. Make it your goal to drink at least 1.5 to 2 litres of tap (filtered or distilled if possible) water or mineral water each day. Use a BPA-free water bottle so you can easily measure and monitor how much water you drink. Herbals teas without caffeine can also count toward your goal.

Navigating the Supermarket (and More)

When negotiating the supermarket, stay out of the middle — shop the perimeter! You find most of the natural food that you should load up on — meats, fish, eggs, vegetables, fruits and dairy products — along the outer perimeter of the grocery store. Processed and packaged foods generally make up a majority of the shelves in between. With the exception of nuts, legumes and oils from the aisles, most of the selections in your shopping cart should consist of whole foods from the store's outer ring.

Making your list and sticking to it

Planning your meals in advance is a vital part of eating well and avoiding reactive eating. An integral part of executing your plan is maintaining your grocery list. Without the right supplies, you'll have a hard time providing quality nutrition for yourself and the rest of your family.

On your grocery list, keep a running list of all the items you need for the upcoming meals that you've planned. List some healthy snacks to have on hand too. Don't forget to include healthy beverages like sparkling water, mineral water and green tea. Double-check the pantry for any ingredients you need for recipes, and be sure that you have enough staples like extra-virgin or cold-pressed olive oil, butter, herbs, teas, coconut shreds, organic cans of legumes, sardines, tuna and spices on hand for cooking.

When planning menus and making your grocery list, try to include local vegetables in a variety of colours. Different colours indicate different phytonutrients, so make an effort to include red, green, orange, purple and white vegetables (see Table 6-1).

Table 6-1	Fruit and Vegetable Colour Chart
Target Colour	*Example Foods*
Red vegetables and fruits	Tomatoes, red capsicum, red onions, raspberries, strawberries, cherries, radishes
Green vegetables and fruits	Spinach, rocket, silverbeet, fennel, leeks, celery, lettuce, green beans, broccoli, brussels sprouts, Asian greens, green capsicum, watercress, zucchini, cabbage
Orange/yellow vegetables and fruits	Yellow capsicum, oranges, mandarins and tangerines, pineapple, lemons, carrots, papaya, butternut pumpkin, sweet potato, kumara
Purple/blue vegetables and fruits	Beets, blueberries, eggplant, currants, plums, purple onion, grapes, purple cabbage
White vegetables and fruits	Cauliflower, pears, garlic, mushrooms, onions, parsnips

Table 6-2 shows some simple substitutions you can make on your grocery list to improve the quality of your food.

Table 6-2	Simple Grocery List Substitutions
Instead of This	*Buy This*
Commercial minced beef	Grass-fed minced beef or lamb
Soft drinks	Mineral or sparkling water
Sweetened bottled drinks: teas, 'vitamin waters', flavoured milk	Green, rooibos, licorice or cinnamon tea bags
Seasoning packets	Fresh herbs, garlic, chilli, ginger, lemongrass, mint, cumin, turmeric, sea salt, pepper, lemon rind
White rice	Brown rice or quinoa
Peanut butter with sugar and hydrogenated oil	Natural peanut butter, ABC spread (almond, brazil nut, cashew) or any nut butters
White bread or Turkish bread	Spelt, rye, pumpernickel or wholegrain bread
White pasta	Brown rice pasta, spelt pasta or corn pasta

Reading and understanding food labels

The nutrition facts label is your key to uncovering the truth about the food inside. The nutrition facts label shows you the serving size, the kilojoule count, the basic nutrition breakdown (protein, carbs, fat, sugar, sodium and so on) and, most importantly, the ingredients. An example of a typical nutrition facts label is in Figure 6-1.

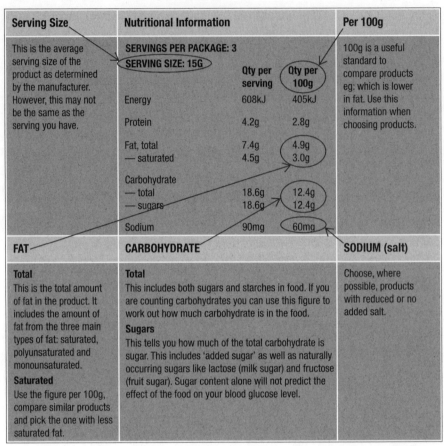

Serving Size	Nutritional Information			Per 100g
This is the average serving size of the product as determined by the manufacturer. However, this may not be the same as the serving you have.	**SERVINGS PER PACKAGE: 3** **SERVING SIZE: 15G**			100g is a useful standard to compare products eg: which is lower in fat. Use this information when choosing products.
		Qty per serving	**Qty per 100g**	
	Energy	608kJ	405kJ	
	Protein	4.2g	2.8g	
	Fat, total	7.4g	4.9g	
	— saturated	4.5g	3.0g	
	Carbohydrate			
	— total	18.6g	12.4g	
	— sugars	18.6g	12.4g	
	Sodium	90mg	60mg	
FAT	**CARBOHYDRATE**			**SODIUM (salt)**
Total This is the total amount of fat in the product. It includes the amount of fat from the three main types of fat: saturated, polyunsaturated and monounsaturated.	**Total** This includes both sugars and starches in food. If you are counting carbohydrates you can use this figure to work out how much carbohydrate is in the food.			Choose, where possible, products with reduced or no added salt.
Saturated Use the figure per 100g, compare similar products and pick the one with less saturated fat.	**Sugars** This tells you how much of the total carbohydrate is sugar. This includes 'added sugar' as well as naturally occurring sugars like lactose (milk sugar) and fructose (fruit sugar). Sugar content alone will not predict the effect of the food on your blood glucose level.			

Figure 6-1:
Nutrition facts label decoded.

© Diabetes Australia

Even though most of your healthiest meals consist of whole foods without labels, you should watch out for trouble on the nutrition labels of anything you buy that comes wrapped or boxed — bread, crackers, cakes, pies and condiments, for example.

Here are several things to watch out for on nutrition labels:

✔ **Enriched flour:** Even baked goods that prominently display *whole-wheat* or *whole grain* on the packaging are often made of mostly enriched flour, with just a sprinkling of wholegrain flour added in. Read the ingredients list to see whether the primary flour is enriched flour, and look for products with organic wholegrain flours as the first ingredient instead.

✔ **High sugar content:** Educating yourself on the added sugar on a nutritional panel may take a bit of detective work. Manufacturers are required to put the amount of sugar per serving on the nutritional label for products sold in Australia and New Zealand, but they don't have to make it clear how much of that sugar is added sugar. If sugar or some form of sugar is in the first three ingredients, know that the product is most likely high in sugar. Replace any packaged food with more than 5 grams of sugar per 100-gram serving with a healthier choice. Be on the lookout for ingredients that appear in the 'Other names for sugar' sidebar earlier in this chapter. Check out the sidebar 'Reading between the sugar lines' for more on making sense of the sugar content in food.

✔ **Total carbohydrates:** Look at how many grams of carbs are in each serving. This includes starches, complex carbs, dietary fibre, added sugar sweeteners and non-digestible additives. The following add up to the total carbohydrate value:

   • **Dietary fibre:** This amount represents the amount of fibre in each serve, in grams. We recommend 25 to 30 grams of fibre per day.

   • **Sugars:** The number of grams of sugar here includes added sugars and natural sugars, like lactose from milk and fructose from fruit.

✔ **Trans fats:** If you see the word _hydrogenated_ anywhere in the ingredients, put the item back on the shelf.

Pay attention to the serving size noted on the nutrition label of packaged foods. Measure out a serving to see how that compares to the amount that you normally eat; you may find that without checking, you ordinarily eat two, three or even four servings' worth of calories and sugar!

Reading between the sugar lines

When looking at the sugar and carbohydrate content on food labels, here are a couple more things to consider:

✔ The total carbohydrates listed on the label minus the sugar content listed can be helpful in figuring out what percentage of the food is made up of sugar. For example, All-Bran cereal contains 24 grams of total carbs and 6 grams of sugar, leaving 18 grams of healthy carbs. However, if a soft drink label has total carbs of 40 grams and total sugar of 40 grams, you know 100 per cent of the carbs are coming from sugar, not complex carbs — in other words, the soft drink gives you zero healthy carbs.

✔ To give yourself a quick visual of the amount of sugar in a food product, divide the total sugar number by four — this gives you the number of teaspoons of sugar in the product. For example, in a soft drink that has 40 grams of total sugar, dividing this number by four gives you ten — so you can now imagine ten teaspoons of sugar being poured into the bottle you're looking at. Yikes!

Eating local: Farmers' markets

The grocery store isn't the only place where you can find healthy food. Farmers' markets offer great opportunities to get fresh, organic, locally grown foods. Actually meeting the farmers who deliver food into your community is an easy way to ascertain the origin of your food (and to verify the farming methods used to produce it) and to become more actively involved in your own nutrition. Doing so also provides a great opportunity to teach your children the importance of being proactive about healthy eating.

You can visit www.farmersmarkets.org.au/markets and www.farmersmarket.org.nz to find farmers' markets, family farms, community-supported agriculture organisations, and other sources of organic and sustainably grown food in your area.

3-in-1 healthy meal planning

Our clients often state that the primary reason they don't eat better is that they don't have time to cook every day. If you struggle with finding time to cook, this 3-in-1 meal planning system may be just the trick! The basic idea is that you cook once and then use whatever you made for two (different) subsequent meals. So this isn't just cook once eat twice — now we're advocating eat at least three times! For example, prepare grass-fed beef tenderloin for dinner one night, and then use the leftovers for sandwiches and stir-fry on subsequent days. Here are some more examples using chicken and salmon:

3-in-1 Chicken

✔ Day 1: Roast a chicken (rosemary with vegetables is a favourite).

✔ Day 2: Use the leftover chicken to make a Mexican enchilada by wrapping it up with some sautéed onions, melted cheese, sour cream, and lettuce and tomato. This takes less than five minutes to make.

✔ Day 3: Pull the remaining chicken off the bones and sprinkle it in a mixed green salad.

3-in-1 Salmon

✔ Day 1: Cook a big piece of wild-caught salmon (you can use the Grilled Salmon with Coriander Salsa recipe in Chapter 15). Serve it with a side of green beans sprinkled with olive oil and sesame seeds.

✔ Day 2: Make salmon cakes! (See www.ahealthyview.com.au or adapt the Too Easy Salmon Cakes recipe from Chapter 15.) With a side salad of baby spinach and avocado you're sure to be satiated!

✔ Day 3: Make salmon stir-fry by adding the remaining salmon to fresh veggies and wild rice in your favourite sugar-free sauce. Your vegetable chopping time is only a minute or two, and the cooking time is only six minutes.

Considering pasture-raised meat

Regardless of whether you decide to buy organic produce, if you eat meat we recommend that you choose pasture-raised beef and chicken. Animals that are pasture-raised are much healthier because they have access to their natural diet and get plenty of exercise and sunshine. Animals raised in conventional feedlot operations are confined to overcrowded pens where, instead of their natural diet, they may be fed genetically modified grains and given large doses of antibiotics.

As you may imagine, an animal's diet has an enormous impact on the nutritional content of the meat from that animal. Scientific studies show that regular consumption of feedlot meat causes inflammation and increases the risk of heart disease and cancer. Grass-fed meat, however, has been shown to have less fat, higher vitamin and mineral content, a healthier ratio of omega-3 to omega-6 fatty acids, and higher concentrations of conjugated linoleic acid (CLA), a cancer fighter. Meat isn't bad for you — *bad* meat is bad for you!

Organic beef isn't the same as *grass-fed beef.* Organic meat comes from animals that are raised without antibiotics and are fed an organic vegetarian diet (which may or may not include corn and grains). Grass-fed beef is meat from cattle raised solely on grass, hay and forage.

Going Sugar-Free on a Budget

In general, whole food is more expensive than packaged food, and organic food costs more than industrial food products. The popularity of clean organic food is bringing the price down over time, but at present, sugar and chemicals are unfortunately still cheaper than quality food. You can take some steps, however, to make sugar-free or low-sugar nutrition more affordable.

Stretching your grocery dollars

If you find yourself on a tight food budget, here are some tips to get the most for your money without resorting to junk food:

- ✔ Check local newspapers, grocery and supermarket websites, and coupon sites for in-store specials and discounts. Ask about a loyalty card for extra savings at stores where you shop. Meat and seafood are often the most expensive items on your list, so when you find a good deal, buy extra and stock the freezer.

✔ Other than items you can freeze, don't buy too much food at one time. Produce and fresh meat only keep for a few days in the refrigerator, so don't buy more than you can use in the next few days.

✔ Don't shop when you're hungry! Stick to your list, and try to be at the grocery store or supermarket when you're not too rushed so you can make smart decisions.

✔ Check the 'use-by' dates and be sure that you pick the freshest option. Grocery stores don't always rotate stock reliably.

✔ Instead of deciding on a meal and then buying the ingredients for it, try reversing the process and seeing what healthy meals you can invent using what you already have in the house.

✔ Stretch expensive meats into more portions by using them in meals like stews, casseroles and stir-fry.

✔ Buy produce locally in season — it's not only less expensive but also fresher and a better environmental choice.

Knowing when to buy organic

Our preference is to buy organic food whenever possible. Not being exposed to pesticides, herbicides, chemical fertilisers and genetically modified plants is worth the extra money. Plus, it's important for society to support farmers who use chemical-free, environmentally responsible methods. The more we support these types of practices, the less expensive they will become for us.

Understandably, not everyone is willing or able to commit to organic food full-time. Sometimes your food budget may require that you buy less-expensive conventional produce instead of organic foods. If that's the case, don't worry — the benefits of a diet that's high in vegetables and fruits outweigh the risks from pesticide use and genetically modified food. If you have to prioritise, go with organic when you buy foods that have been shown to accumulate high concentrations of pesticides. The following is a list of the top 20 Australian foods with the most pesticide detection (2000 to 2011):

✔ Apples (15.2 per cent)

✔ Wheat (13.2 per cent)

✔ Strawberries (10 per cent)

✔ Pears (9.5 per cent)

✔ Grapes (6.4 per cent)

✔ Lettuce (4.1 per cent)

✔ Nectarines (3.7 per cent)

✔ Peaches (2.3 per cent)

- Bread (2.1 per cent)
- Bran (1.8 per cent)
- Biscuits (1.6 per cent)
- Tea (imported) (1.6 per cent)
- Barley (1.4 per cent)
- Tomatoes (1.3 per cent)
- Apricots (1.2 per cent)
- Canola (1.1 per cent)
- Flour (1.1 per cent)
- Carrots (0.8 per cent)
- Plums (0.8 per cent)
- Green beans (0.8 per cent)

The preceding list comes from data collected by Friends of the Earth — go to www.foe.org.au/sites/default/files/TheDoseMakesThePoisonFeb2012_0.pdf for more information.

The following lists the foods in New Zealand found to have the most pesticide residues (ranked according to number of pesticides detected in total samples and percentage with pesticides):

- Celery (98.2 per cent with residues; 21 pesticides detected)
- Peaches, fresh/canned (96.4 per cent with residues; 15 pesticides detected)
- Apricots, fresh/canned (96.4 per cent with residues; 14 pesticides detected)
- Butter/cream/cheese (100 per cent with residues; 3 pesticides detected)
- Wheat: bread, all products (79.3 per cent with residues; 23 pesticides detected)
- Apples (80.5 per cent with residues; 20 pesticides detected)
- Plums (91.6 per cent with residues; 8 pesticides detected)
- Mandarins (83.3 per cent with residues; 10 pesticides detected)
- Raspberries (85.4 per cent with residues; 7 pesticides detected)
- Oranges (82.1 per cent with residues; 9 pesticides detected)
- Strawberries (71.1 per cent with residues; 16 pesticides detected)
- Grapes/raisins/sultanas (57.1 per cent with residues; 25 pesticides detected)

The preceding list comes from data collected by Organic NZ — see http://www.organicnz.org.nz/node/120 for more information.

Rinsing reduces but doesn't eliminate pesticides. If you use lemon rind, which we recommend for flavouring in your salads and vegetables, purchase organic options or grow your own lemons. Peeling removes more chemicals but also removes valuable nutrients along with the skin. Buying organic is the best option, if possible. If you think you can't afford organic, perhaps think about what you're spending your income on — long-term wellness or short-lived material things.

Chapter 7

Sugar Detox Made Easy

· ·

In This Chapter

▶ Understanding the myriad benefits of a sugar detox

▶ Getting started on your detox journey

▶ Checking out complementary medicine therapies and practitioners

· ·

*D*etox and *cleanse* are two terms that are often used to indicate a dietary plan that reduces or eliminates consumption of unhealthy substances. Whether you take a step-by-step approach to gradually reduce your sugar intake or you quit sugar cold turkey, you'll reap the benefits of detoxifying your body from the harmful effects of sugar overload.

This chapter helps you appreciate all the mental, physical, emotional and medical benefits of getting off sugar — many of which you may never have thought of. We also give you a few tips on finding some holistic medicine options that may assist your quest to detox from sugar.

Appreciating What a Sugar Detox Can Do for You

Sugar, in excessive amounts, is one of the most harmful substances you can eat. When you look at lollies, soft drinks, pies, cakes and flavoured milks, you may not think of the word *toxin,* but refined sugars (along with other artificial sweeteners) place a huge physiological stress on your body's systems. High blood sugar levels cause damage to blood vessels and organs, and high insulin levels promote fat storage. Sugar makes your immune system less effective and creates a strong inflammatory response throughout the body. And while all of that is going on physically, your hormones, energy, mood and emotions are becoming equally unbalanced. Getting off sugar can end all that!

Detoxing from this inflammatory substance gives you a jump-start down the road toward weight loss, improved energy, better immune system function and superior nutrition. A simple sugar detox can also quell your cravings for sweets, improve your mental clarity, and lead you toward a more empowered and fulfilled life.

CEOs, educators, doctors and countless other participants in Michele's programs have told how moving to a low-sugar way of eating has changed their life, their work and their relationships with people. One of Australia's business leaders told Michele he didn't realise what an impact his blood sugar had on his productivity until he came off what he referred to as his 'sugar hits'. He unashamedly now says he never misses a meal and keeps a stash of protein-based, low-carb snacks on hand to munch on before important meetings and phone calls.

Read through Chapter 3 for an understanding of sugar and carbohydrates and how to avoid hidden sources of sugar.

Is going cold turkey best for you?

We generally advocate a gradual approach to sugar reduction because a drastic, overly-strict eating regimen isn't a sustainable system for most people. However, we do occasionally encounter an individual for whom a rigid, cold-turkey approach to quitting sugar works best. Only you will know your personality type and if you can handle the fast, furious nature of cold turkey. Or, perhaps you require the slow, gentle approach. Neither is right or wrong; it is what works for your body.

If you decide to stop eating sugar cold turkey, treat yourself like you're in detox for an addiction to narcotics. The first week of sugar abstinence is the hardest because that's when the cravings are the most powerful. Be gentle with yourself in other areas of your life — this isn't the time to tackle a large project, implement lots of other life changes, or work overtime. Give yourself extra support by going to bed early, taking naps when you need them, taking long baths or meditative walks, and cooking simple, nourishing meals. Call on others for support and encouragement when you need it (see Chapter 11 for advice on building a support system).

Aiding weight loss and getting rid of toxins

When you stop feeding yourself empty sugar calories, and when your insulin levels aren't elevated from eating too many carbohydrates, you begin to lose weight. More specifically (and more importantly), you begin to lose body fat.

 Body fat is toxic. *Adipocytes* (fat cells) secrete inflammatory proteins that contribute to cardiovascular disease, arthritis, Alzheimer's disease, vascular dementia, fibromyalgia and other diseases brought on by chronic inflammation. Body fat cells are also storehouses for toxins in your body. Many substances that your kidneys and liver can't metabolise — pesticides, polychlorinated biphenyls (PCBs), and poisonous metals like lead and mercury — are tucked away and stored in fat cells (in the toxicology field, this is referred to as *bioaccumulation*).

Detoxing from sugar gives you a powerful head start toward shedding toxic body fat.

Achieving better blood sugar and insulin control

Excessive sugar or other carbohydrates elevates blood sugar levels and triggers an overproduction of insulin (consult Chapters 3 and 4 for more information on carbohydrates and insulin). Chronically high insulin levels may lead to obesity and diabetes. Detoxing from sugar stops the insulin roller-coaster and helps level out your blood sugar levels, which is critical to avoiding (or reversing) diabetes.

Experiencing increased energy

When your blood sugar levels are stable, you don't experience the post-insulin sugar crashes that cause fatigue and 'brain fog'. Less sugar in your diet helps keep your energy high and balanced, especially if you get some consistent exercise (see Chapter 12 for the lowdown on exercise).

In addition to smoothing out your blood sugar levels, detoxing from sugar indirectly helps coax your thyroid and adrenal glands back to their normal function, so you'll no longer suffer from the overwhelming fatigue that afflicts so many sugar addicts. You can read more about how sugar affects your hormones and endocrine system in Chapter 4.

Getting more nutrients

Sugar, along with many other sweeteners like corn syrup, contains zero nutrients, only calories. When you eat sugar, you consume calories without nutrition, and this leads to weight gain, malnutrition (even if you're overweight) and cravings.

When you start replacing empty sugar calories with higher-quality proteins, fat and carbohydrates like vegetables and fruits, you dramatically increase the amount of essential vitamins, minerals and phytonutrients in your diet. Your body requires these vital nutrients to stay vibrant and to prevent all manner of diseases and illnesses. Better nutrition leads to a healthier body and fewer sugar cravings too! Refer to Chapter 5 for an overview of healthy nutrition basics.

Improving immunity

Dumping a large amount of sugar into your stomach lowers your immune system's effectiveness by about 30 per cent for several hours. Consistent sugar consumption keeps your immune system permanently depressed. A sugar detox allows your immune system to leap back to full function.

Another important component of the immune system is the *intestinal flora*. The good bacteria in your gut stimulate the production of immune cells and play a major role in metabolising dietary carcinogens. A high-sugar diet creates imbalances with your intestinal flora, compromising your immune system and allowing foreign pathogens (like yeast) to flourish. Detoxing from sugar and using a quality probiotic supplement (refer to Chapter 5 for advice on probiotics) restores the intestinal flora to a healthy state. Visit www. ahealthyview.com.au for recommended brands of probiotics and other nutrition supplements.

Reducing inflammation and lowering your risk of disease

The inflammatory response is a necessary part of your physiology. Your body uses controlled inflammation to heal wounds, fight infections and rebuild muscles. But too much inflammation can lead to premature ageing and potentially to major problems such as atherosclerosis, eczema, arthritis, yeast infections, chronic pain, autoimmune disorders, Alzheimer's disease, vascular dementia and cancer.

Sugar is an inflammatory food, so if you eat sugar frequently you're placing your body in a continuously inflamed state. If you don't yet suffer from inflammation problems, getting off sugar now can help prevent the possibility of some terrible diseases in the future. If you're currently battling one or more inflammatory conditions, detoxing from sugar will lower the inflammation in your body and help relieve some of the discomfort of irritable bowel syndrome, Crohn's disease, fibromyalgia, gout, arthritis and other conditions caused by chronic inflammation.

Having less gas

Sugar creates an acidic environment that harms the beneficial bacteria in the gut. Your body's good bacteria (the intestinal flora) are important for digestion, immune system function and serotonin production.

Eating too much sugar alters the intestinal flora, and the sugar ferments in the intestines, leading to bloating and gas. Cutting back on your sugar intake reduces gas and diminishes that uncomfortable, bloated feeling.

Battling fewer cravings

Consistent sugar overdose wreaks havoc on your brain chemistry (refer to Chapter 2). If you're a sugar addict, the more sugar you eat, the more you want. Breaking the craving cycle is a big step in changing your eating habits for the better. As you start to wean yourself off sugar (or if you quit it cold turkey), you'll find that within a very short period (usually two to four weeks), you no longer desire sweet foods. And if you do have some sugar, you'll find that the sickly-sweet goodies you used to dream about don't even taste good anymore.

To start overcoming your sugar cravings right away, flip to Chapter 9 to investigate identifying triggers and to start using the step-by-step guide for what to do when a craving strikes.

Enjoying better skin

The inflammation from a high-sugar diet makes your skin prone to unsightly pimples, eczema and other breakouts. Sugar also damages collagen, causing your skin to become stiffer and less elastic. The more sugar you eat, the more tissue damage you may cause and the more wrinkles you get. Staying away from sugar is one of the best things you can do for your skin.

Michele recently heard from a client who, after following a low-sugar plan for six weeks, was losing weight. The customer then explained how everyone wanted to know where she was getting her new botox injections. She was proud to say that the amount of weight she was shedding was nothing compared to how glowing her skin looked. And she'd had no injections of any kind!

Sharpening mental clarity

In addition to physically damaging your brain, a sugar binge can cause a host of brain performance problems. Sugar addicts commonly suffer from a sugar 'hangover', with symptoms like brain fog, fatigue, headaches or emotional swings.

Detoxing from sugar stops the sugar highs and crashes, keeping your energy more stable and your brain more functional throughout the day. You'll sleep better too!

A strong link has been found between sugar and dementia. A study that appeared in the *Journal of Neurology* found that people with impaired glucose (not even diabetes) were 35 per cent more likely to develop some type of dementia. So detoxing from sugar also has long-term benefits, and may help you avoid a very sad battle.

Feeling personal empowerment

One of the most powerful and life-changing rewards of beating sugar addiction (or any addiction) is the thrill of empowering yourself and running your life proactively, so that you're in charge of your own behaviour. To make a blanket generalisation, addicts tend to use external substances to supply them with the brain chemistry they desire. When you detox from whatever substance you've been using as a substitute for a healthy emotional state — in this case, sugar — you'll live a happier and more peaceful life, and your body will thank you for healing it after sugar's harmful onslaughts.

When you overcome sugar addiction, you take a giant step towards creating or improving other positive things in your life — relationships, exercise, career issues, time management and self-care. When you start taking control of your attitude and your actions instead of living reactively from the stresses of the world, food hangovers and negative thoughts around food, there's no end to the wonderful things you can accomplish for yourself and for others!

Taking Your First Detox Steps

Sugar detox is simply the act of stopping the ingestion of harmful amounts of sugar so that your body can begin to heal itself by de-acidifying your blood and tissues, shedding excess body fat, and coaxing your hormone and energy systems back to normal, healthy function.

Follow these tips to ensure success when you begin detoxing from sugar:

- ✔ **Create a list of reasons you want to live differently.** Common reasons are to become healthier, to regain control of your life, to overcome diabetes, to have more energy or to lose weight. But you may have other personal reasons for quitting sugar. List the *whys* and not the *shoulds* — to stay on track, it's very important to have personal, meaningful reasons for wanting to change.

- ✔ **Cut your sugar portions in half each day until it's fully eliminated.** Unless you really need to quit sugar cold turkey, start a gradual sugar reduction plan by cutting your typical sugar intake in half. For example, if you eat two fruit yoghurts per day, go to one. If you have a sports drink per day, reduce it to only half the bottle until you get to none.

- ✔ **Drink at least 1.5 to 2 litres of water each day.** Water helps keep sugar cravings at bay and means you don't confuse thirst for hunger (refer to Chapter 5).

- ✔ **Eliminate sugar from your pantry and refrigerator.** You can't eat what you don't have! Keeping your household free of junk food makes it difficult to impulsively grab sugary snacks. Consult Chapter 6 for tips on performing a healthy kitchen makeover.

- ✔ **Redefine dessert.** Until you have made a full transition to low sugar and can trust yourself, have desserts that aren't typical 'sweet desserts'. Naturally sweetened herbal teas, like Black Adder or Cinnamon Apple, are replacements for sweets. When you feel you are in complete control of your addiction, usually a bite or two of fresh fruit or dark chocolate (70 per cent cocoa or more) satisfies your desire for something sweet at the end of a meal. See Chapter 17 for low-sugar dessert ideas.

- ✔ **Start getting some regular exercise.** A good workout burns calories, increases your energy, boosts your mood, tones your muscles, and increases your bone density and insulin sensitivity. Go to Chapter 12 for tips on setting up a basic exercise program.

- ✔ **Stay away from sweetened drinks.** Sweetened beverages are a huge source of empty calories (refer to Chapter 3), and diet drinks made with artificial sweeteners carry some significant health hazards. Make water, tea or mineral water your drink of choice.

Using Complementary Medicine for More than Just Detoxing

Because a lifetime of sugar abuse can cause significant damage to the body, some sugar addicts struggle with serious medical conditions resulting from years of an abusive diet. Improving your diet and getting some regular exercise are great first steps toward improving your health, but you may consider widening the scope of your health improvements to include stress management, personal growth and holistic medical care. Our patients commonly begin to feel good without sugar and then want to take this new sense of wellbeing further into their lives.

Despite their sincere desire to assist in the wellbeing of their patients, general practitioners (GPs) often don't have the time, or necessarily the knowledge, to pass on nutritional education. GPs can prescribe medications to treat lifestyle diseases, but you may get more comprehensive advice about preventative measures — such as improving your health through nutrition and lifestyle changes — from nutritionists and other complementary medicine practitioners. *Complementary medicine* (sometimes called *integrative medicine* or *holistic medicine*) is a catch-all term used to describe a method of patient care that combines conventional Western medicine with complementary treatments such as nutritional education, nutrition supplements, acupuncture, massage therapy, yoga and stress-reduction techniques.

Complementary therapies and modern medicine are merging rapidly as some of the world's leading hospitals are combining hospitals, clinics and research centres into integrative care facilities. New York's Sloan Kettering Memorial Hospital (a renowned cancer research facility) and Stanford Hospital are just two examples of integrative medicine complementing mainstream care.

Regardless of the practitioner you're seeing, you need to take responsibility for your own health. Your GP, your trainer, your nutritionist and your specialist can't own your health — only you can! Build a support network of educated practitioners (see Chapter 11), keep all your own records and notes, and take personal responsibility for creating the lifestyle habits that will keep you (and your family) healthy. Discovering a more well-rounded system of medical care can get you started in the right direction and multiply the benefits of your sugar detox.

Big pharma's influence on your doctor

Sometimes traditional GPs unfairly get a bad rap because of the poor track record that Western medicine has concerning improving the health status of its patients (refer to Chapter 4 for more on the rise of obesity, diabetes and health-care costs). In our experience, most GPs are well-intentioned (although time-poor) professionals who do their best to help their patients using the training they've received and the time they have.

Many doctors aren't receptive to (or educated about) non-pharmaceutical treatments. But bear in mind how influential pharmaceutical companies are becoming. Because they are so profitable, drug companies fund many of the research published in the major medical journals and pay speakers at medical seminars. A report by the US Consumer Reports National Research Center surveyed more than 1,150 adults who currently take prescription drugs and found that the vast majority object to the incentives and rewards pharmaceutical companies routinely give to doctors, because they feel these are negatively influencing how they treat their patients.

Exploring complementary medicine options

Complementary medicine strives to treat the whole person, not just the disease symptoms. Examples of some integrative medicine therapies that have proven to create positive patient outcomes are:

- Acupuncture
- Biofeedback
- Chiropractic
- Exercise programs
- Health coaching
- Massage therapy
- Meditation and mindfulness practice
- Mind–body therapies
- Naturopathic medicine
- Nutrition counselling
- Tai chi
- Yoga

Integrative medicine is no longer considered fringe because it has been shown to be a success in medical centres that have implemented it within their systems. The number of hospitals that now offer complementary therapies has more than tripled in the last ten years, and another quarter of hospitals say they plan to add complementary therapies in the future.

Finding a synergistic practitioner

If you're interested in making a concerted effort to maximise your physical and emotional wellness, detoxing from sugar is a good first step. But you can do much more. To make good overall health a top priority, you need to seek out doctors and other advisors who understand more than just the standard practices and ideologies of traditional medicine. Fortunately, you can find plenty of doctors and other health-care providers who consider a wide range of treatments and health enhancements that aren't limited to prescription medications. Some GPs specialise in nutrition and complementary therapies, and some nutritionists integrate themselves with GPs. In our opinion, this synergist combination is the future of preventative medicine.

The following section provides some help with finding a quality integrative practitioner.

Using judgement and seeking recommendations

Just like any GP or specialist, some good alternative health practitioners are available, as well as some not so good ones. A quick internet search for any medical condition yields a host of results for miracle cures, quick fixes, and testimonials, often without a shred of research or clinical practice to back up those claims. You need to vet complementary and alternative medicine (CAM) practitioners and products carefully because bogus practices and products can be not only a waste of time and money but also downright dangerous. Consider the following:

   ✔ **Avoid any therapy that promises that it's the only solution or cure to your problem.** Quality integrative medicine doesn't blindly advocate a single alternative approach while rejecting all conventional ones. If the practitioner or product you're investigating promises to be the be-all, end-all to your problem and automatically dismisses all conventional treatments, move on. A quality integrative practitioner will be happy to work on your condition with other professionals such as a GP or a psychologist. If they're not, move on.

✔ **Ask your trusted friend, general practitioner, physical therapist or other health-minded individual whom you trust for a recommendation for the type of provider you seek.**

✔ **Check with peak bodies for a list of reliable complementary practitioners who are qualified and have insurance.** In Australia, check with the Australian Traditional Medicine Society (www.atms.com.au); in New Zealand, go to the Nutrition Society of New Zealand (www.nutritionsociety.ac.nz).

✔ **Use caution with 'food coaches'.** Food coaches are advisors on food, health and nutrition, but aren't nutritionists. They can't offer treatment for specific health conditions and haven't undertaken the years of study and training that a diploma or degree requires. So make sure your choice — food coach or qualified nutritionist — is correct for your needs.

✔ **Consult a qualified nutritionist before choosing nutrition supplements or powders.** Some nutrition supplements can have serious side effects or interactions, and the purity and labelling accuracy of nutrition supplements varies widely among manufacturers. To be sure you have a safe and effective nutrition regimen in place, you really need to consult with a knowledgeable professional, not someone behind a counter making a commission on what they're flogging to you.

Part III
Living a Successful Sugar-Busting Lifestyle

Meal	Planned Eating Time?	Protein?	Complex Carb (i.e. Veggies)?	Quality Fat?	Hydration Adequate?	Energy Level After Eating?
Greek yoghurt, seeds and blueberries	6.30 am	✔			✔	✔
Handful of nuts with green tea	10 am	✔			✔	✔
Turkey wrap	1 pm	✔	✔		✔	✔
Wholegrain rice cracker with almond butter	4 pm	✔	✔		✔	✔
Grilled fish and sautéed veggies	7 pm	✔	✔		✔	✔

Illustration by Wiley, Composition Services Graphics

Discover key tips and special secrets to avoid holiday 'Silly Season' weight gain at www.dummies.com/extras/beatingsugaraddictionau.

In this part . . .

- ✔ Master mindful eating to control your portion distortion and enjoy your eating experience.

- ✔ Identify triggers that send you reaching for sugary foods.

- ✔ Know what to do when a craving strikes and sort out what your body really needs instead of sugar.

- ✔ Keep in mind simple tips when eating out at restaurants, parties and special occasions.

- ✔ Surround yourself with a reliable support system and be prepared for how people may react to your change in lifestyle and eating habits.

- ✔ Increase your chance of success by including an exercise plan with the right balance of cardio and strength training.

Chapter 8

Eating Mindfully

● ●

In This Chapter

▶ Explaining the concept of mindfulness

▶ Engaging in proactive eating

▶ Using strategies to cultivate a consistently mindful approach to meals

● ●

*1*n counselling thousands of clients over the last 20 years, we've found that one theme reigns supreme: People have a hard time living purposefully instead of reactively because they feel that their lives are busy and often out of balance. This mindset can lead to a host of stress and anxiety disorders like sleep problems, weight gain, headaches, thyroid disease, panic attacks, autoimmune disorders, heart attacks and cancer.

Chinese medicine has a word for this frantic, out-of-control mindset — *xinyuan*, which translates, wonderfully, into 'monkey mind'. The term was adopted into Buddhist and Confucian teachings more than 1,500 years ago, but it has also become a popular term in modern psychology.

An uncontrolled monkey mind is the antithesis of a peaceful, happy and calm life. It's a serious detriment to your health and wellbeing, and will wreak havoc on any dietary planning you attempt. To regain control of your life, you must learn to master your monkey mind.

Mindfulness is the key to quieting the monkey mind. This chapter lays out an explanation of mindfulness and how it relates to controlling your eating. We deliver tips on eating with intention and planning, and avoiding being obsessive about food. Our goal in this chapter is to give you a mini course in living proactively instead of reactively so you can use those tools to create a healthy, sustainable eating plan to help you stay healthy, lean and craving-free forever.

What Is Mindful Eating?

Mindfulness is the act of being mentally and emotionally present, without judgement, while being aware of and intentional about your state of mind and your behaviour. Basically, it means paying attention to what's happening without judging or reacting, and acting purposefully and intentionally. (Judging often means your judgement on yourself — we are our own worst critics.)

Mindful eating requires that you pay attention to the cues your body gives you. It's easy to become fooled or distracted by external events, unhealthy habits and unskilful reactions to the hiccups along the road of life.

As you learn to pay attention to cues from your body, and as you practise making food decisions intentionally instead of reactively, you'll regain control over your eating style, and the careful attention and purposeful decisions will carry over to other aspects of your life. Mindful behaviour of any type is a gateway to a more peaceful and empowered life!

Mastering Proactive versus Reactive Eating

Turning to food, especially sugar, when you feel stressed or out of control is very easy. Sugar is pervasive in most of the world, and this cheap, readily available drug can exert harmful control over your life if you let it.

Keep away from the 'CATS' — coffee, alcohol, tobacco and especially sugar — when you feel tired and stressed.

Proactive eating means that you don't allow external cues to affect your eating behaviour (what you choose to eat, when you eat and how much you eat). Proactive eating decisions come from knowledge, planning and consistent practice. Eating proactively is a skill that you must master to achieve lasting weight loss and to kick the sugar habit for good.

Here's a scenario that typifies unhealthy, reactive eating: After a long, stressful day at work, you come home late, too tired to cook something healthy for dinner. You plop down in front of the TV and begin munching on a bag of whatever you can grab out of the pantry. While you eat and watch, you also go through the mail, worry about this month's bills, and try to decide what you're going to wear to an event this weekend that you don't really want to go to anyway (mostly because you don't feel good about yourself). When the bag is empty or when you feel disgusted with yourself for what you just ate, you finally stop eating. In an hour, you're hungry again because you haven't eaten properly, but because you've already 'fallen off' and eaten the wrong foods, you think you may as well just continue eating the 'treats' you keep for a special occasion.

Examine some of the unmindful points of this scenario:

- You didn't plan ahead; dinner was an afterthought, and you ate whatever was handy. The pantry and freezer were stocked with unhealthy fast-food kilojoules.

- You paid no attention to the amount of food you ate. You can't control portions when you eat directly from a bag.

- You paid no attention to your body's cues. When you eat from a bag while doing several other things, you have very little awareness of any physical sensations or emotions. You have no idea when you've had enough to eat or why you're doing what you're doing.

- You didn't focus on any one task. The monkey mind stayed in full force the entire evening.

Here are some easy ways to improve the mindfulness of this situation:

- Eat well during the day so that you're not starving when you get home.

- Keep your kitchen stocked with healthy food instead of convenience calories (refer to Chapter 6).

- Plan the day's food so that you don't have to think about what you're going to eat for each meal. Planning is the key.

- Put your food on a plate before you start eating and take an honest look at what's there. Do you have vegetables? Where's your protein? What are the portions like? What's this meal going to do to your insulin levels? Can you improve what's on that plate without too much trouble?

- While you're eating, savour the tastes and textures. Chew thoroughly. Pay attention to how your body feels so you know when you've had enough. The Japanese use the term *hara hachi bu*, which means 'stomach 80 per cent' — in other words, stop eating when you're 80 per cent full.

- Stay focused on one task at a time. While you're eating, pay attention to that and only that. When you're engaged in a conversation with a friend, colleague or child, focus on that conversation. Texting while having a conversation is just adding to your monkey chatter. When planning for future things, do so one at a time, using facts and strategy instead of reacting to anxiety and worry.

Paying Attention While You Eat

The practice of mindfulness is concerned with noticing (without judging) what's happening *right now*. That doesn't mean you can't think about the past or the future, but when you do, you should strive to do so without fear or judgement, and you shouldn't allow recognition of past events or future fears to dictate your behaviour in the present.

Staying mindful is a skill that requires attention and practice. Without focus and attention on the present moment, the mind wanders to thoughts of the past or to worries about the future. This triggers all sorts of negative emotions like fear, anger, guilt, depression and self-pity. If you indulge these kinds of thoughts, you reinforce their power in your life and the habits that you've built around them — most likely sugar abuse, if you're reading this book.

Eating with intention

Eating purposefully (instead of reactively) is the most important skill for controlling your weight and staying away from sugar. The lifestyle of modern society has created a host of external food cues that can easily override your body's natural cues about eating. While eating, instead of deciding whether they're still hungry, people typically use external cues to tell them when to stop. For example, an empty dinner plate is an external cue that it's time to stop. For most people, even if a few bites of muffin remain in the wrapper or if a few soggy chips are left at the bottom of the bag, they unconsciously decide that they must continue eating. People habitually eat as though their mission is to finish every last bite in front of them, because they were often forced to do this as children.

To stay mindful while you're eating, evaluate how you feel after every bite. Are you 80 per cent full yet? Are you experiencing what you're eating or just chewing and swallowing mindlessly? What does what your food actually taste like if you were describing it to us? Are you eating because you need nourishment or are you eating as a reaction to something external: Being annoyed at your partner, a child, a co-worker? Are you reacting to not enough sleep?

Here are some tips to help avoid mindless eating situations:

- ✔ **Don't eat out of packages.** Put your portion on a plate or in a bowl and put the package away. If it's in front of you, you'll most likely eat it until it's gone. Portion it, place it and walk away.

- ✔ **Don't put serving dishes on the dinner table.** If you want more food, make yourself get up and go into the kitchen to get it.

- ✔ **Keep food out of sight.** Food that's visible (sitting out or in a glass container) gets eaten more, because every time you pass the lolly jar at the office, you have to make a decision about whether to eat some. Every time you see it, you have to say 'No' to something tasty and tempting. Eventually, the 'No' turns into, 'Well, okay, just this once . . . ' Use 'out of sight, out of mind' to your advantage.

- ✔ **Enjoy your food in a calm setting.** Watching TV and eating can lead to mindless eating. Enjoy your food with family and friends.

- ✔ **You don't have to eat everything that's on your plate.** When you have more than protein and vegetables on your plate, don't feel obligated to eat it all. It may seem wasteful at first, but in the future you will tend to place less on your plate. (Think about whether you'd prefer to be wasteful or waist-full.) You can also potentially save leftovers for lunch.

Planning your food choices in advance

Many people fall victim to reactive eating because they're unprepared. If you don't know in advance what your food will consist of for the day, you're at the mercy of the cravings of your starving brain, which will drive you to grab whatever you can get quickly — and lots of it!

Eating on the fly with no plan is akin to investing in a company that has no budgets, where everybody says, 'We just spend whatever we feel like from day to day and hope it will all work out in the long run. Then we complain about how broke and cranky we are.'

Plan your eating in advance, out to whatever time horizon suits you. Most of the people we know who really strive for good health and wellness plan their next day's food the night before, and some prefer to lay out a week at a time so they only have to think about it once a week. Any time frame that works for you is fine, as long as you don't leave the house without knowing what you're going to eat for every meal and snack for the rest of that day.

Planning should include not only *what to eat* but also *when to eat* and *how much to eat*. Plan your eating times in your schedule as much as possible — doing so keeps you from going too long without food and succumbing to cravings and ravenous reactive eating.

Planning portions is easy if you prepare your own meals and snacks, but it can be tricky if you eat out a lot. The good news is if the majority of your food is coming from protein and vegetables, you can be assured that it will be low sugar. At restaurants, avoid using the empty plate as the only measure of whether you're finished eating. Look at the plate when it arrives and assess your portions using the list from Chapter 5. Eat vegetables first, then protein. After that, assess your 80 per cent — do you need the extra carbs or any more kilojoules? Probably not.

Here are some factors to consider when planning your meals:

- ✔ Do you have protein and quality fats in the mix? Refer to Chapter 5 if you need help with protein and good fat sources.

- ✔ Do you have complex carbs and vegetables at this meal? If you're bringing a sandwich for lunch, make sure it's loaded up with fresh lettuce, tomato, onion, beetroot, capsicum, or whatever other veggies you like.

- ✔ Have you considered your portions? Remember, no eating from packages or serving dishes. If you're planning on eating out, be aware of your portions before you take the first bite.

- ✔ What will this meal do to your blood sugar? Refer to Chapter 3 for information about your carbohydrate choices' effect on your insulin response. This is especially important if you have diabetes.

Use the handy chart in Figure 8-1 to double-check your plan for the upcoming day, and help you assess how you're feeling after the meal. After listing the meal or snack and the time you plan to eat it, the chart has five columns for you to check off.

Meal	Planned Eating Time	Protein?	Complex Carb (i.e. Veggies)?	Quality Fat?	Hydration Adequate?	Energy Level After Eating?

Figure 8-1:
Use this chart to plan ahead for meals.

Keeping a food journal keeps you honest

A food journal is one of the best tools for staying mindful and honest about how much, how often and what you're actually eating. After you eat something, write it down straightaway. At the end of a busy day, trying to remember what you had at what time (and how much of it) is asking for inaccuracy, denial and selective memory. You should record every single thing that goes in your mouth, including water. If you bite it or drink it, you write it! You may do this for a few months and then it becomes habitual, and you may not need a journal.

Research shows that people who really want to make a change and keep a food journal lose more weight than those who try to improve their eating without one. In our experience, people tend to think they eat better than they actually do. When you record a few days of consumption, you may find that you're woefully short on vegetables or that you regularly eat way too many calories before bed. One bonus to keeping a food journal is that it makes you think more about what you choose and how much you eat. People generally report that keeping a food journal automatically improves their eating just by virtue of the fact that they have to think about it and write it down. Your journal doesn't have to be complicated; in fact, the simpler it is, the more likely you are to use it.

Visit www.ahealthyview.com.au to download a basic food journal and to look over the recommended reading list for additional resources and guidance toward better mindfulness.

Avoiding being obsessive or neurotic about food

Being mindful and educated about what you eat isn't the same as being obsessive or neurotic about food! Making smart choices from an informed and empowered position is desirable, whereas making decisions out of fear or deprivation can lead to guilt, resistance, overcompensation and even eating disorders.

Food isn't your enemy, and you can't build a successful, healthy eating plan if you consistently act out of fear or resentment. To tell yourself that you'll never eat sugar again is unrealistic. Being aware of hidden sugars is your aim. Your goal should be to be better, not to be perfect. Any food plan that uses the word 'never' is destined to lead to trouble and often a rebound.

Obsessing over every tiny detail of your diet, being a control freak and trying to be perfect are behaviours that stem from the fear of a lack of ability or personal power. Every time you find yourself at a decision point, remember that you're the decision-maker and the driver of your destiny. Empower yourself to make positive decisions in all phases of your life, and don't allow a fear of setbacks to drive you to an obsessive or neurotic view of food.

Friends can provide an enormous amount of support on your quest to eat better (see Chapter 11), but obtaining assistance from a trained professional is often helpful. If you'd like to receive some professional help with mindful eating or if you have concerns about obsessive eating habits, consult the Australia & New Zealand Academy for Eating Disorders website at anzaed.org.au for information and treatment referrals. Also visit The Butterfly Foundation www.thebutterflyfoundation.org.au.

Summoning willpower and understanding

Many people who struggle with sugar and weight control try to change their ways through fad, deprivation or strict diets, thinking that willpower is what they need. When their unsustainable plan goes awry, as it inevitably does, they tell themselves that they've blown it and give up completely.

From a mindfulness perspective, you never reach a point of no return; you can choose to eat mindfully at any time, even after blowing it for one meal or even for a whole month. People occasionally make choices they're not proud of. Own what you did (no excuses; it was your choice), recognise the effects that those behaviours have on your body, and make a plan to do something different next time. Don't keep putting yourself down over it — just move on to positive steps.

Willpower is useless without an understanding of what you really want (see Chapter 9 for an important lesson about that). If you try to deny yourself the sugar that you're craving without stopping to think about why you're craving it, you'll eventually give in to the brain's cravings. And you'll have learned nothing and changed no behaviours or habits.

Willpower is sustainable when you use it as the discipline to get organised (and stay organised) and to act (and eat) purposefully and mindfully instead of reactively. If you bank on willpower to keep you away from sugar when you don't have planning and mindfulness in place, it will fail you.

Managing stress

One of the most reliable paths to sugar addiction and obesity is high stress, because stress changes your appetite, stimulates overeating and increases insulin resistance.

Surveys show that a majority of women often eat for emotional reasons rather than hunger. Stressful emotions dampen the reward response in the brain and stimulate cortisol, which causes cravings that drive overeating (and, for some people, the abuse of other substances too). Stress affects the same signals as famine does: It turns on the brain's pathways that make people crave calorie-dense food (high fat and high sugar). The hunger and reward drives are some of the strongest in the human body, and they're very difficult to combat without the right tools.

Learning to turn the monkey mind into mindfulness is a lifelong practice, but here are a few simple stress-management tips that can get you started:

✔ **Breathe.** Stopping to take a few deep belly breaths gives you a moment to gather your thoughts and become rational. (We mean really breathe, taking conscious full breaths.)

✔ **Empower yourself.** Remember that you're the one driving the bus. If you don't like where it's going, drive somewhere else! Don't be someone who finds someone or something else to blame. If you create a solid nutritional foundation and hold yourself accountable, you can find a sense of empowerment. One of our favourite quotes from famous self-help author Wayne Dyer is, 'Remember that you choose your attitude and your personality every second of every day.'

✔ **Find meaning in what you do.** If your job is causing you stress, remember what you liked about your job when you started it. Consider what you may need to do differently to be satisfied in your position again. Think about the necessity of your work, the purpose of your job, your personal goals and the benefits that your work provides to others.

✔ **Identify the true source of your stress.** Stress comes from fear, so when you find yourself feeling overwhelmed or stressed out, take a moment to determine what you're afraid of. After you give yourself a reality check, you can determine whether your fears are well-founded. If they are, you can start taking appropriate action instead of just worrying.

✔ **Schedule something that you like to do that's just for yourself.** Take a walk, get a massage, read for fun or have a nap. Taking time for yourself is not selfish. If you replenish yourself doing something good for you — a nourishing activity and/or nourishing food — you will find that you will be a better friend, partner or parent. Be sure to put the activity on your schedule or you'll never get to it!

In Chapter 9, we help you identify triggers and choose substitute behaviours.

Giving yourself a reality check

Becoming overwhelmed by a busy life is easy if you don't regularly pause for a reality check. Staying mindful helps you understand what's actually happening, what you're really afraid of and what you really want.

When you find yourself faced with a negative emotion like anger, stress or a sugar craving, ask yourself these three questions:

✔ What actually happened just before I reacted the way I did? Just the facts here — no blaming, assuming or history allowed!

✔ What story am I making up (or what belief do I have) that led me to create the emotion I'm having?

✔ What other attitude or emotion can I choose instead of a negative, unfriendly one?

One of the greatest stress relievers is to uncover what a particular stressor or incident really means to you. For example, if you're feeling stressed out about work because you think you can't get everything done, ask yourself what not getting things done means to you. Does it mean that you're a failure? Do you think it means that you're unappreciated or misunderstood? Does it mean that you're unreliable or unlovable?

Shining the light of truth on your fears can uncover their blatant untruths or at least make them less scary.

If you haven't yet taken the quiz in Chapter 2, do so now and see whether one of the four typical behaviour and psychology profiles fits your situation. Understanding the whys of your thoughts and behaviours helps keep your head on straight and gives you a powerful tool to stay on track with healthy eating habits.

An experiment in mindful eating

To get a feel for how mindful eating can enhance your eating experience, try this sequence the next time you're ready to sit down to eat something that you love. The first few times our patients do this they often feel uncomfortable — like they're trying to be someone off a cooking show — but try the process at least once. Doing so really helps you eat mindfully. We love scrambled eggs with smoked salmon and rocket so we use this as an example:

1. Before you do anything else, stop and be grateful for what you have and for what you're about to do.

2. Savour the smell and enjoy the visual aspects of your meal before you have your first bite.

3. Place a forkful in your mouth. Think about the temperature, texture and initial taste.

4. Now comes the hard part — put the fork down. This is more challenging than you may think because that first bite feels and tastes so good, and the rest of the plate is

calling you. You're hungry, after all! This experiment in eating, however, involves looking past the instinctive urge to vacuum the rest of the eggs up. Leave your fork on the table.

5. Chew slowly. No talking. Savour the flavours.

6. When you've chewed thoroughly and taken in all the new sensations you can for now, go ahead and swallow your first bite.

7. When you've finished savouring, pick up your fork and take another bite. Continue this way throughout the course of the meal and you will practise mindful eating.

The concept of mindfulness has its roots in Buddhist teachings. Paying close attention to the sensation and purpose of eating, your interactions with people and your general daily activities expands your consciousness and appreciation. If you enjoyed this mindfulness experience with food, try practising more mindful awareness during a walk after dinner!

Chapter 9

Staying On Track with Your Low-Sugar Plan

. . . .

In This Chapter

▶ Adopting new mindsets and new habits

▶ Working out what makes you crave sugar

▶ Getting on top of cravings

▶ Taking the right steps when you fall off the wagon

. . . .

*N*o-one should be expected to sustain an eating plan with zero fulfilling or enjoyable foods, and that includes you. Food and mealtimes are meant to be enjoyed. This chapter talks about how to develop new habits and new ways of dealing with food without trying to remain on an unsustainable, restrictive 'diet' (we really dislike that word!). We help you find your new normal, that all-important mindset that guarantees you'll never again feel like you're on a diet. In fact, remove the word *diet* from your world, because it conjures up *restriction*. Instead, embrace this 'new norm', which offers such delicious, healthy alternatives that you won't even think about the unhealthy foods you left behind.

Habits can be hard to change, and you won't always be perfect. If you're depressed, tired or stressed, you may find yourself craving sugar or falling back into other unhealthy habits. This chapter helps you forgive yourself, deal with your inner critic, and get back in the driver's seat after a bad choice. Don't beat yourself up. Sure, hiccups can occur along the path, but if you keep with your eating plan for the long term, the lifestyle just becomes routine. If you fall off the rails, restart at your next meal.

To avoid those hiccups in the future, this chapter also shows you exactly what to do when a craving strikes — a step-by-step system for staying on track!

Applying Strategies for Success

Everyone is different, but after helping more than 1,000 people overcome sugar addiction, we've identified some clear patterns. This section examines must-do strategies for success — vital skills to achieve the new habits and new mindset you'll need to successfully break the cycle of sugar addiction.

As you pick up these principles and progress down the path of mindful eating, not only will you have more energy and feel much better, but your tastes will probably change. After usually two to four weeks of low-sugar eating, your desire for sweet things is likely to drop dramatically! Two patients of Michele's emailed her shortly after they did a sugar cleanse. Initially, they had slowly reduced sugar, then had a one-week residential, no-sugar cleanse and then continued for a third week in their own homes. After approximately 21 days, they attended a friend's 40th birthday party where they had their first glass (since the cleanse) of much-loved champagne. They were so overwhelmed with the sugary taste they asked the host if he had put some sugar syrup into their champagne!

Adopting a new mindset

Any aspect of your life — your body, your relationships, your friendships, your attitudes — is strongly influenced by what you do most of the time. Whatever is 'normal' for you yields a certain result. If you want to change some part of your life, you have to change what you usually do — you have to create a *new normal*.

Changing what's normal for you

Take a moment and write a sentence or two that describes what's currently normal for you in each of these circumstances:

- ✔ Breakfast
- ✔ Choice of snacks
- ✔ Eating frequency
- ✔ Food portions
- ✔ Late-night eating

- ✔ Planning your food (versus eating on the fly or eating whatever's handy)
- ✔ Vegetable intake
- ✔ Quality fat and protein intake
- ✔ Water intake versus other drinks
- ✔ Stress reaction
- ✔ Sleep habits

The goal of any successful eating plan is to create a healthy, sustainable normal so that you're never on a diet or on a special plan; you just do things differently from how you used to do them. Improve your normal, and eating well will soon be just something that you naturally do.

Read over what you have written for the exercise in the sidebar 'Changing what's normal for you'. Can you see whether some of your old habits are sabotaging your physical, mental and emotional body? Don't beat yourself up about these habits. Instead, open your mind to seeing yourself in full control and following a new 'normal' for you. For many people, mindful eating seems to be one of the most challenging parts of revamping an eating plan, so you should expect to put some extra effort and attention into eating with purpose instead of reactively (Chapter 8 is all about eating mindfully).

When you find yourself craving something sweet (or when you have the urge for late-night snacking), check in with yourself to see whether food is what you're really after. Are you thirsty? Are you bored? Are you lonely, tired or sad about something? You may find that you've established a habit of wanting something sweet anytime you feel *anything!*

Another big aspect you need to look at is whether you're eating enough. That may seem like an odd aspect to consider with regard to craving sweets but eight out of ten of our patients would admit they're not eating enough quality fat, fibre and protein to keep them truly satisfied. Keep a note of your sugar cravings and look back to see if you properly nourished yourself the meal before the craving hit you. Often people will have an 'Aha!' moment here and recognise they have skimped at lunch only to find themselves ready to break into a vending machine at 4 pm.

You may feel as if needing to include quality fats, fibre and protein in your meals means you're eating too much but trust us — nutrient-dense food that's low in sugar isn't going to pile on the weight. Food that's high in sugar will!

One more important thing to investigate for your new mindset: You have to start looking at how you view food. How do you respond to the following questions? (**Remember:** No judgement is present here — this book is between you and the honest you.)

- Do you view food as your friend (maybe your only friend)? Your enemy?

- Do you use food as a reward? How about as a substitute for affection or mental stimulation? Have you been medicating yourself with sugar?

Here's your new mindset: Food is nourishment. It's fuel for your body. You truly are what you eat. You need to start seeing food as nourishing fuel. Eating should also involve an enjoyable, social aspect. However, if you're unconsciously sabotaging yourself, and you use food as an unhealthy substitute for something else you need, food begins to hold a very dangerous power.

Spend some time thinking about what stories you may be making up about sugar. For example, 'I need this hit of sugar in my tea and a bit of chocolate to get me through the afternoon.' 'I have had a wicked day and I deserve this ice-cream; it will soothe me and I will restart tomorrow.' 'It's cold out; I need sugar to warm me up.'

Hmmm, maybe instead of the sugar hit you need to get more sleep, have a bath, enjoy a nourishing bowl of chicken soup, or talk to a friend for some real nourishment.

Developing new habits

Sometimes the idea of changing your daily routines can seem daunting. When we talk to new clients, they often report that in the past they felt overwhelmed by all the things they thought they had to keep track of when they tried to improve their eating habits. Don't despair! Developing new habits isn't as complicated or overwhelming as it may seem. Don't try to change everything at once, and don't think that from now on you have to eat perfectly all the time and deprive yourself of your favourite foods forever!

The following sections cover three essential yet simple habits you can adopt to stay on track with a quality eating plan.

Decide what and when to eat instead of eating reactively

The biggest challenge most people face is eating *purposefully* instead of *reactively.* To get off sugar and eat healthfully for the rest of your life, you need a new mantra: Decide to be proactive, not reactive! You don't have control over some of the things life throws at you — for example, a car accident, ill children, retrenchment from a job or other curly life situations — but when you're in a nutritionally sound balanced body, you can manage these situations a whole lot better.

If you lose control over your food intake every time something unexpected or stressful happens in your life, you'll never be able to sustain a healthy eating system.

Plan ahead with three meals and two healthy snacks

Planning ahead is one of the most important habits you must develop to eat purposefully. 'But I'm time poor', you say? Ask yourself this: Have you truly accomplished anything in your life without planning? A new business, a sport, a craft — they all take time and planning. Why wouldn't you plan for your health, your most valuable asset? Before you go to bed each night, take a minute and go through your meal planning for the next day. Write it down at first, especially if you find that you feel overwhelmed with planning meals in addition to everything else on your to-do list. Planning is the key to your success. At first this will take time but as it becomes your new 'normal' it will be a daily process not requiring much fuss. Make sure that you're prepared for the day's eating schedule with this checklist:

✔ **Protein-packed breakfast:** A breakfast high in protein helps control your blood sugar levels and staves off hunger more than a breakfast of all carbohydrates (cereal, muffins, banana bread, toast and so on). A protein-packed breakfast might include eggs, antibiotic-free breakfast meats (sausage or ham), a 'clean' whey protein shake, or some Greek yoghurt. For more in-depth information on protein, refer to Chapter 5. You can find breakfast recipes in Chapter 13.

✔ **Morning tea:** To keep blood sugar levels stable and to avoid cravings, your morning snack should include protein. Examples are an apple with almond or peanut butter, a small handful of almonds or walnuts, a slice of cheese and some grainy crackers, a cup of cottage cheese, or hummus with some raw vegetables. Refer to Chapter 3 for more information about blood sugar control and Chapter 16 for yummy, low-sugar snack recipes.

✔ **Lunch:** Don't forget to load up on the veggies at lunchtime! Here are a few good lunch examples:

  • A chicken or tuna sandwich or wrap with wholegrain bread and lots of green lettuce, avocado, tomatoes, spinach, beetroot, onions or whatever other veggies you like. To minimise the amount of bread, try an open-faced sandwich with just one slice of bread. Or you can make a 'roll hole' by digging out the fluffy bread in the middle of a roll to make more room for your protein.

  • A mixed green salad with grilled salmon and lemon vinaigrette dressing. Use up the leftover salmon from your previous evening's meal for this salad.

  • Mixed vegetables and diced chicken sautéed in olive oil.

  You can find more low-sugar lunch ideas in Chapter 14.

✔ **Afternoon tea:** Your afternoon tea should be like your morning snack (that is, it should contain protein), but try to vary it a bit. Many people find that something with a desirable 'mouth feel' helps keep them satisfied during the afternoon. If you like creamy, try plain Greek yoghurt. If you like crunchy, try some apple slices or celery sticks with a handful of almonds.

✔ **Dinner:** Be sure to have a healthy dinner planned, so you're not grabbing unhealthy foods when you come home hungry after a long day. Having fresh fish or a chicken breast ready to cook allows you to put together a healthy, speedy meal. See Chapter 15 for some delicious dinner recipes.

Dinner should be your lightest meal of the day — and, if you've fed yourself appropriately throughout the day, this should be easy. If all you plan to do after dinner is watch TV and go to bed, you don't need many kilojoules! When you eat too much food before bed, you don't have a chance to burn off those kilojoules, and they're simply stored as body fat.

In addition to the list of what you're going to eat, make sure you have

- ✔ Plenty of filtered or sparkling water to drink throughout the day.
- ✔ Any other approved sugar-free beverages you desire, like mineral water with citrus, or herbal teas like green, rooibos, lemongrass, cinnamon or licorice tea. Teas can taste nourishing, especially if the weather is cool.

Obey the ten-minute rule

When a craving strikes, always wait ten minutes before acting on it. The ten-minute rule gives you time to decide on something smarter to eat, gives you a few minutes to distract yourself with a positive substitute activity (see 'Choosing substitute behaviours' later in the chapter), or allows you the opportunity to figure out what you really want besides food. Perhaps make yourself a cup of tea and ask yourself if you're thirsty, tired or bored? Or, you simply may be hungry and ready to eat.

Making a gradual transition versus going cold turkey

As you change your mindset and your eating habits to reduce sugar, you can experiment with two different approaches. One is to work through a gradual transition in which you phase out sugary foods and make selective substitutions over time. The other approach is to quit sugar cold turkey.

Some people have better success making a gradual transition away from sugar. A slow transition to healthier eating is often easier on the family too. This is definitely the case if someone in the family is resistant to improving his or her eating habits. Our suggestion is to get yourself 'right' before quietly transitioning your family. (For more on getting your family on board with your efforts to beat sugar, turn to Chapter 11.)

As with most transformations, seeing big changes can take time. For a gradual transition to the low-sugar lifestyle, pick one change from the following list to make each week or two. Soon you'll find that you've transitioned your eating from reactive sugar-grabbing to purposeful, healthy choices.

- **Plan ahead by always bringing a snack to work instead of grabbing whatever's available in the break room or vending machine.**

- **Spice things up.** Adding spices can help in making plain protein-rich meals truly flavourful. For this new lifestyle to be sustainable, you need to really enjoy what you're eating. Become a label reader of bottled sauces and condiments, and begin to substitute high-sugar options with low-sugar alternatives. You don't need to go hunting to a specialty store — the world is becoming increasingly sugar aware, and plenty of low-sugar options are out there, even on the shelves of supermarkets. Check the ingredients — if sugar is not in the first three ingredients, this is a good start. Salsa, spices, sauces and pastes are key in turning your quality protein into a tasty, exciting meal. (Refer to Chapter 6 for more on reading nutrition labels.)

- **Say no to soft drinks.** Soft drinks equal lots of kilojoules without any nutrients. Don't be fooled by diet soft drinks, either — they're known to stimulate sugar cravings. Make unsweetened tea or mineral water with fresh citrus instead.

- **Cook once, eat twice.** Make enough low-sugar dinner to provide leftovers for lunch the next day. That way you're not at the mercy of trying to find something healthy when buying a takeaway option — which can be full of hidden sugar and expensive.

- **Pick a weekend day when you and your family cook everything from scratch.** It's fun, it's quality family time, and you'll have lots of healthy food ready for the rest of the week.

- **Make an effort to try to buy fresh or frozen foods rather than canned or processed foods.** If you need to purchase canned or processed foods then become a label reader. What is in the list of ingredients, what is the serving size, and how much sugar does it contain? (Refer to Chapter 6 for more on reading nutrition labels.)

- **Start cutting back on white-flour starches and start adding more vegetables.** Foods like white breads and pastas, bakery treats and croissants are low in nutrients and fibre and high in kilojoules and carbohydrates. Try replacing white-flour products with wholegrain or non-wheat choices like brown rice, wholemeal pasta, quinoa or sweet potatoes. (Refer to Chapter 6 for more on avoiding white-flour products.)

Our recommendation for most people is to attempt a gradual transition to a no/low-sugar lifestyle if at all possible. However, some folks do better just going cold turkey — cutting out their sugar intake completely in one fell swoop. If you know yourself well enough to know that the only way for you to break the cycle of sugar addiction is to quit sugar completely, here are some things you can expect:

✔ **Your family may not want to transition with you, and that's okay.** Get yourself through your nutritional transformation first and then consider taking family members down this path with you. When others see you transforming, the changes they see in you will create a butterfly effect. Hopefully, other family members will become inquisitive and transition with you. If they don't, don't get caught up in their story. Stay with your own story — the journey to good health.

Enthusiastic sugar celibates can become overzealous. We have witnessed this amazing, healthy change countless times and, because people just feel so good, they want to take everyone on this ride with them. Super-successful businesspeople Michele has worked with often remark that they didn't even know that they were feeling average until they started to feel so energised and de-bloated — and they then employ her to present to their whole company. Enthusiasm is good and understandable, and we love sharing this new-found energy. Just keep in mind that not everyone is ready for a change.

✔ **You may be tired for the first week or two.** You may feel like you have the flu. Over the years of addiction, you've likely taught your system to rely on sugar and caffeine for energy, and now you're asking your body to step up and function normally without these substances and without any notice or preparation. Stick with it; it gets better soon! Be kind to yourself during this time with naps, baths and quiet time. Recalibrate.

✔ **Your appetite will change.** Some people report that they're much less hungry after they stop eating sugar. Why? Because your insulin receptors can come alive again. Glucose and nutrients can now get into your cells, giving your smart body a satiated sensation. Your appetite changing usually takes a month, so be kind and consistent with yourself.

✔ **You'll stop craving most sugar after you've been clean for a week or two, and your cravings will truly wind down after four weeks.**

✔ **Regular, healthy food (like vegetables) will taste better and be more flavourful to you.** After you've retrained your taste buds (and your brain) to be accustomed to a normal level of stimulation, you can start really tasting food's flavour. Some of Michele's clients say they now find having something with sugar in it unappetising.

If quitting sugar cold turkey sounds like the best approach for you, learning to eat mindfully will help you with the process — check out Chapter 8 for instructions and advice.

Shopping with purpose

Unless you grow and raise all your own food, mindful grocery shopping is an integral part of staying prepared and purposeful. A simple grocery list that you keep handy (Dan leaves his out on the kitchen counter) is a very important planning tool. When you see you're close to running out of an item, write it down. Before you go to the supermarket or the farmer's market, think about the next few days of eating. How many protein servings do you need? How much produce? Do you have snacks ready? Write it all down on the list. It sounds simple, but remember that you have to have a plan ready to execute. Otherwise, you won't be prepared and you can easily fall back on reactive, mindless habits. Not planning ahead is one of the things that has kept you stuck in your sugar-loving lifestyle until now!

Here are some other grocery shopping tips to help you succeed in cutting sugar:

- ✔ **Don't shop when you're hungry.** When your blood sugar is low, you go into survival mode and can lose the ability to make good decisions.

- ✔ **Focus your food shopping on the outer perimeter of the store — produce, meats and seafood, eggs and dairy.** Most of your food should come from the perimeter. Most of the processed food that's loaded with sugar and chemicals is located in the centre aisles.

- ✔ **Don't buy tempting junk food 'just for the kids' or 'just for my partner'.** If you haven't planned well and it's in the house when you're starving, you're going to be in trouble. Your family shouldn't be eating that stuff anyway! Fill your pantry and refrigerator with so much quality food that your family doesn't even realise their junk food isn't there.

- ✔ **Stick to your list!** Don't take home enticing impulse buys that may be poor food choices and also expensive.

Unravelling Those Overwhelming Sugar Cravings

Sun Tzu, the great military strategist, advised, 'Know thyself, know thy enemy'. This couldn't be better advice as you work toward freeing yourself from the enemy of sugar addiction. You must figure out why you've been fooling yourself all these years, and you must understand why you've fallen victim to the false lure of unhealthy eating.

Though this section isn't intended to feel like it belongs in a psychology book, it's important for you to understand the genesis of your sugar cravings and uncover what you really need instead.

Understanding why cravings occur

In a nutshell, sugar cravings are chemical reactions or learned emotional responses (or sometimes both) that typically originate from one of these common situations or conditions:

- **Abrupt weight loss:** A common condition that triggers a physiological sugar craving is losing weight too quickly (commonly the result of crash dieting). Your body has chemical sensors that trigger an alarm if calorie intake drops too low or if fat storage drops too quickly, and the brain turns on the craving centre to replace those calories. Aim to lose weight slowly, or in stages. George Blackburn of Harvard Medical School argues you should aim to lose about 10 per cent of your body weight at first, and then stop. Instead of trying to lose more weight, your focus should be on maintaining your new weight for a while (about six months), giving your body time to adjust to this new normal.

- **Emotional need for serotonin:** *Serotonin* is one of the feel-good hormones, and it gives you that warm, fuzzy, satisfied (and sometimes sleepy) feeling. Serotonin is converted from *tryptophan*, found in protein-rich foods. Sugary foods stimulate insulin, which transports the amino acids — except tryptophan. Instead, tryptophan gets to hang around the brain and convert serotonin. A person with low serotonin will be inclined to consume greater amounts of sugar in an attempt to increase serotonin production. This may lead to sugar addiction.

- **Hormonal fluctuations:** Before menstruation, oestrogen is low and, as progesterone falls, women's endorphin levels are at their lowest. Monthly hormonal fluctuations can explain why many women who experience strong PMS symptoms also have strong sugar cravings — the low endorphin levels may cause them to seek out the serotonin burst that a sugar overload can provide.

- **Inadequate nutrition:** If your diet is deficient in certain nutrients and high in hidden sugars, your blood sugar will peak and plummet like a roller-coaster. During the plummeting lows, your brain seeks out nutrients to get back into a healthy blood sugar range.

Unfortunately, when you're experiencing this blood sugar dip, you might be unprepared and so hungry that you grab the closest (and not necessarily healthiest) option — and off you go again on to a sugar peak and plummet. You need to not only get your blood sugar in balance to stop the cravings but also consume a variety of foods, because your body requires a variety of vitamins and minerals. For neurotransmitters like serotonin, your body requires B-vitamins and magnesium. The best way to get the required variety of nutrients is to eat a range of whole foods that are not processed or packaged! Check out Table 9-1, later in this chapter, for more on nutrient deficiencies and what foods they may cause you to crave.

✔ **Learned behaviour to mask loneliness, boredom or self-deprecation:** As mentioned earlier, sugar equals serotonin. If you're feeling bad, eating sugar can temporarily make you feel better. It's very easy to learn how to substitute unhealthy eating habits for introspection and personal work. When the inner critic starts scolding you, an easy way to quiet the critic is to drug yourself with sugar. The same goes for when you're feeling lonely, bored or anything else you don't particularly like to feel. Instead of doing the hard personal work that's required to change their ways of thinking and interacting with the world, many people take the easy way out and ignore their problems by zoning out with sugar (or sometimes, even worse, drugs).

✔ **Stress:** When you're under stress you produce *cortisol*, a hormone that can increase your feelings of hunger. Cortisol is your body's reaction to a 'fight or flight' situation, where your body goes into survival or emergency mode. In this survival mode, you need a quick source of energy, and sugary foods can give you that. Unfortunately, in the Western lifestyle, people aren't burning up the sugar they eat in response to stress, because their stresses are more emotional and mental, and not the same as their physical ancestors who were hunting and killing for survival.

Filling the void: What do you really want?

Abstinence will not keep you off sugar for good. In order to successfully beat sugar addiction, you must change your relationship with food by finding wisdom at the root of what is incomplete in your life.

We always encourage clients to really dig deep into their alleged desire for sugar. Although introspection and self-discovery are lifetime pursuits, the following sections introduce some basic concepts that may help you become more self-aware right away.

Ask what you really need

When you have an urge to grab something sweet, stop for a moment and answer these questions:

✔ Am I hungry?

✔ Am I tired?

✔ Am I thirsty?

✔ Am I bored?

✔ Am I lonely?

✔ Am I feeling bad about myself or about something else?

✔ Am I overwhelmed or feeling stressed?

Chances are you want something besides sugar. Once you have identified the real issue, you can start to find ways to satisfy what you really need instead of medicating yourself with sugar.

Look at the circumstances that preceded the craving

People are creatures of habit. If you start to look for patterns in your cravings for sugar, chances are you will notice that when certain things happen, your brain turns on the craving centre. Next time you have an unhealthy craving, look at the circumstances that preceded it. Here are some situations that commonly precede a sugar craving:

✔ When you don't sleep well

✔ When you haven't eaten a proper meal for a while

✔ When you feel overwhelmed at work

✔ When you feel unloved by your spouse

✔ When you feel out of control about a family situation

✔ When you haven't had enough water

✔ After you've eaten too many carbs, and not enough protein and fat

✔ When you're worried or anxious about something

✔ After you've eaten too much

✔ When you can't find anything interesting to think about or to create

✔ When you begin obsessing about what treats you think you're missing

✔ When you feel like you want to reward yourself

If you notice a consistent pattern of cravings after one or more of these situations, change or attend to the situation or condition that precedes the craving! One of the easiest ways to beat sugar cravings is to avoid or fix the situations that trigger them in the first place. Don't play in traffic!

Letting your craving tell you what's missing from your nutrition

Cravings can often be a signal from your body that you're missing some important nutrients. Table 9-1 shows some possible correlations.

Table 9-1	Nutritional Deficiencies That Can Cause Cravings	
If You Crave or Have This	*You May Be Deficient In*	*Get What You Need from These Foods*
Chocolate	Magnesium	Bran, raw nuts and seeds, legumes, spinach
Toasted bread	Nitrogen	High-protein foods (fish, meat, eggs)
Fatty or oily foods	Calcium	Dark greens (spinach, mustard, turnip, kale), broccoli, cheese, yoghurt
Chewing ice	Iron	Red meat, poultry (the dark pieces), seaweed, greens, raisins
Burned food	Carbon	Fresh fruits and vegetables
Carbonated drinks	Calcium	Dark greens (spinach, mustard, turnip, kale), broccoli, cheese, yoghurt
Salty foods	Chloride	Fish, sea salt, goat's milk
Acid foods	Magnesium	Bran, raw nuts and seeds, legumes, spinach
Preference for liquids instead of solid food	Water	Flavour with fresh citrus if you like
Avoidance of liquids in preference of solid foods	Water	You've been dehydrated for so long that your thirst centre has melded with your hunger centre; drink small amounts (100 mls) of water every one to two hours throughout the day
Pre-menstrual cravings	Zinc	Red meats, oysters, root vegetables

(continued)

Table 9-1 *(continued)*

If You Crave or Have This	You May Be Deficient In	Get What You Need from These Foods
Ravenous appetite (without having gone too long without food)	Silicon	Bananas, green beans, oats, whole grains; avoid white 'enriched' flour
	Tryptophan	Dairy, plain yoghurt, lamb, turkey
	Tyrosine	Avocado, almonds, orange and red vegetables and fruits
	Dietary fat	Fish oil, first-pressed olive oil, flaxseed oil, coconut oil, cheese
Lack of appetite	B-vitamins	Meats, eggs, seeds and legumes, grains
Sweets	Chromium	Onions, tomatoes, oysters, whole grains, broccoli, grapes, mushrooms, reputable multivitamin/mineral supplement if required (always try food first)
	Magnesium	Bran, raw nuts and seeds, legumes, spinach, green leafy vegetables

Managing Cravings

Even after you've started to change your thinking, your habits, and your food content, your sugar cravings won't disappear overnight. Unlearning old habits and old ways of thinking is a process, and while you work on improving your ways of eating and thinking, you're bound to experience occasional sugar cravings. This section talks about things you can do to minimise these cravings, identifies common triggers, and walks you through the exact steps of what to do when a craving strikes.

Timing your meals properly

In order to keep your blood sugar levels stable and ward off emergency cravings for energy, eating often is important. A good rule to remember is to eat a combination of protein and complex carbohydrates every 3 to 4 hours. If you go longer than that without eating, your body goes into 'starvation emergency' mode and starts holding on to its fat stores and cranking up the appetite centre. By eating small amounts of quality food every few hours, your blood sugar levels will stay nice and even all day, and your body will happily use fat as its preferred energy source for your activities.

If you go longer than that without eating a protein source, your body may begin to break down muscle tissue (and organs!) in a process called *catabolism* to replenish the missing amino acids. Any eating habits that cause loss of muscle tissue lower your metabolism.

Following smart nutrition practices

In addition to meal timing, you can use the following nutrition practices to help ward off cravings. If you'd like to dive deeper into these principles, you can find a more detailed look at nutrition in Chapter 5.

- ✔ **Don't confuse thirst for hunger.** Often people who are chronically dehydrated lose their sensation of thirst. The thirst centre in the brain then melds with the hunger centre so many people who are unknowingly dehydrated will get a food craving when what they really need is water. Dehydration also increases fatigue and decreases mental alertness.

- ✔ **Avoid artificial sweeteners.** Aspartame (NutraSweet) is a chemical that is harmful to your brain, and some studies show that it increases appetite. Regularly over-stimulating the taste centres of the brain with artificial sweeteners increases the desire for that extra-sweet taste. If you absolutely must flavour your beverages, use unbleached stevia root powder instead of sugar or chemicals.

- ✔ **Eat enough during the day.** If you skip, you dip. Big drops in blood sugar levels lead to big cravings for sugar and carbs to bring it back up. Sometimes the late-night cravings are a signal that you haven't eaten enough earlier in the day, and your body is looking to make up those extra calories.

- ✔ **Eat lots of vegetables.** Three main reasons that snacking on vegetables can help stave off sugar cravings:

  - Vegetables are high in nutrients and low in calories. *Remember:* A deficiency in certain nutrients can turn on the craving centre.

  - The crunch factor that many vegetables possess can give you a satisfying chewing experience and pleasurable 'mouth feel'. Many sugar addicts (and smoking addicts too) have reported to us that the mouth feel is one of the main reasons they seek out snacking or smoking, so crunchy vegetables can serve as a much healthier option to fill that desire.

- The fibre in vegetables helps you feel full. Research shows that your stomach gets accustomed to a particular volume of food, so you often will not feel satisfied until you have ingested a particular amount of food, regardless of its calorie content. Eating lots of high-volume, low-calorie vegetables will help you feel full without going overboard on the calories.

✔ **Plan ahead.** Remember that most of the 'convenience' food that's available quickly isn't very healthy. Before you leave the house (or even the night before), be sure to plan your eating for the day. Either bring your low-sugar options with you, or have a plan in place for what and where you will eat throughout the day.

Identifying triggers

Triggers are events or situations to which you react. Often in the case of the sugar addict, those reactions are habits that are both learned and chemically induced. In order to consciously change your reactions to triggers, you must first identify that you are reacting to a situation.

Here is a new drill for you to practice:

1. **Every time you have a craving, stop and ask yourself what you're reacting to.**

   Is it hunger? A stressful event? An inconsiderate spouse? Thirst? Loneliness? Tiredness?

2. **Take a moment to figure out what you really want (it's not sugar).**

3. **Ask yourself whether eating sugar is going to give you what you really want.**

Use the examples in Table 9-2 to help get you started with this self-questioning habit.

Table 9-2	Adding a Reality Check to Your Triggers	
What Happened	*What I Want*	*Reality Check*
I have stressful deadlines at work	To feel confident that I will get everything done in time	Will eating sugar give me that confidence?
I am tired	A good eight-hour, uninterrupted sleep	Will sugar give me energy and a pillow?
I feel hopeless	Hope	Will eating sugar give me hope?
I'm lonely	Companionship	Will eating sugar give me companionship?
I feel fat or unattractive	To feel better about myself	Will eating sugar make me feel better about myself?
Something my partner said or did made me feel unhappy or stressed	To feel reassured and reconnected to my partner	Will eating sugar give me that connection?
I'm bored	Something engaging for my mind	Will eating sugar give me something interesting to do?
I feel like my life is out of control	Peace and personal power	Will eating sugar give me peace and power?

Choosing substitute behaviours

Another technique you can use to stay away from sweets is to find a substitute activity to engage in whenever you have a sugar craving. We've found that it is important for people to find activities that they enjoy and that they find meaningful. Doing something good for someone else is a great way to get your mind off sugar! Here is a list of some suggestions:

✔ Take a walk.

✔ Ride your bike.

✔ Grab a digital camera or your mobile phone and go looking for interesting photos to take.

✔ Make a list of things to talk about with your partner, therapist or best friend.

✔ Read something interesting.

✔ Enjoy your pet. When was the last time you took the dog for a long walk?

✔ Phone a friend or family member to catch up.

✔ Look up a long-lost friend on Facebook and say 'Hi'.

✔ Write an apology letter to someone you've wronged.

✔ Find a new charity you like, and send a donation.

✔ If you have a partner, write a love note.

✔ Visit someone in the hospital or in a hospice.

✔ Do a Sudoku puzzle, or play chess or Scrabble on the computer — keep your brain occupied!

✔ Do some exercise — you don't need a gym to jog or do crunches.

✔ Update your bucket list.

✔ Pick something in the house that needs to be fixed or cleaned and attend to it.

✔ Look up a subject that interests you and learn something new about it.

✔ Make a list of movies you want to see or books you want to read.

Acting when a craving strikes

In spite of your best efforts to prevent sugar cravings, you're likely to find yourself facing one eventually. Knowing a few defensive manoeuvres helps ensure that you get past the craving without totally derailing your low-sugar plan — although if you do fall off the wagon, the next section helps you get back on. This section is, in our humble opinion, one of the most valuable parts of this entire book — a step-by-step guide of exactly what to do when a sugar craving strikes!

When a craving strikes, follow these steps:

1. **Drink a cold glass of water or citrus-flavoured mineral water.**

2. **Identify what triggered the craving (refer to the 'Identifying triggers' section earlier in the chapter).**

   Don't allow yourself to have the sweet until you come up with the answer.

3. **Make a conscious decision to eat or not eat the sweet.**

   Remember, you're the boss of your behaviour. No-one makes you do anything. If you decide to eat some sugar, you must own it and do it on purpose — don't make any excuses or point any fingers!

If you decide *not* to eat something sweet, choose one or more of these rewards:

- ✔ Give yourself a (healthy) personal reward! Get a massage, book a bush walk, get your nails done or take a long bath.

- ✔ Tell someone! Call or email a friend, write a blog post or make a Facebook update.

- ✔ Choose a positive substitute activity if you wish (refer to the preceding section).

If you decide to eat something sweet, stick to these rules:

- ✔ You must abide by the ten-minute rule — you have to wait ten minutes before you eat a sugary option. If you still want it after ten minutes and you are hydrated, go ahead.

- ✔ Put the amount you will eat on a plate first — no eating from packages or serving dishes.

- ✔ Try a substitute sweet fix:

  - Green tea or, if you're an Exhausted Addict (refer to Chapter 2), licorice tea or cinnamon tea to help restore adrenal function or your blood sugar.

  - A small portion of a low-sugar fruit like cherries, apple, blueberries, strawberries, raspberries or any berries.

  - Chia seed pudding made with coconut milk, vanilla bean and coconut shreds (see Chapter 17 for the recipe).

  - Ice water sweetened with stevia, lemongrass and ginger.

  - A couple squares of dark chocolate (at least 70 per cent cocoa).

Coping with Falling Off the Wagon

No-one is perfect, and no-one eats perfectly all the time. The good news is you don't have to! The key to long-term success is to learn how to make good decisions on a regular basis and not to get derailed just because you've had a less-than-mindful day.

Starting with forgiveness

Mindful eating is a process, a practice that requires, well, practice! You won't be perfect right off the bat. Being mindful about what you eat doesn't mean being neurotic, obsessive or fearful about food. In order to heal sugar addiction (or addiction of any type), you have to heal the emotional brain that you have taught, unknowingly, to crave something to medicate yourself. Healing isn't easy; you're going to have to do some work in order to stay mindful and build new, healthy habits.

If you make a bad decision, or even if you have a whole day of horrible eating, recognise what you did (no excuses), and then forgive yourself, with the intention that you will do better next time. You're not a failure, a freak or a hopeless screw-up. Due to biology, society and your past habits and behaviours, you have become an addict and you need help. It takes time and practice to undo all that past learning. Cut yourself some slack — no-one's behaviour is perfect 100 per cent of the time.

A big difference exists between recognising a mistake and judging yourself. Scolding yourself only worsens your self-negativity, and triggers the emotional insecurities that drive the desire for comfort food in the first place.

Dealing with the inner critic

We all have emotional hot-buttons, but a loud, abusive inner critic is often the trademark of the substance abuser. For many addicts, medicating with sugar, alcohol or drugs temporarily quiets the inner critic. Work on a healthier way to do that!

If you're like most who struggle with addictive personalities, you probably have a well-developed inner critic — that voice continually jabbering away at you, looking for anything to find fault with. It magnifies small failings into giant ones, chastises you over and over for things long past, ignores the true context and doesn't credit you for any of your successes. Sound familiar?

What does the inner critic want? *It wants to be right.* It wants to find evidence to support the same old stories it always tells you. Imagine your inner critic as an obnoxious person at the office who sits around and does nothing except accusingly point at people and say, 'See? I told you, _____!'

After a bad food choice, your inner critic shouts, 'See? I told you how stupid you are; now you've ruined everything!' Is this true? Are you stupid because you made a bad decision? Have you really 'ruined everything'? Certainly not! Successfully beating sugar is a series of ongoing decisions, and you blew one of them. Big deal. You'll get it right next time.

Getting back on track: Three easy steps

Because success with low-sugar eating is an ongoing series of small decisions, when you make a bad decision, being able to get back to making smart ones right away is important. Follow these three easy steps and you'll be right back on the wagon!

1. **State what you did without judging, exaggerating or catastrophising.**

   Just the facts, ma'am. Examples might be, 'I ate the entire banana cake for morning tea', or 'I ate six Tim Tams.'

2. **State why you did it.**

   This one is hard, because you have to look past any story that you told yourself and reveal the truth. The story might be, 'I didn't have time to eat something healthy.' The real truth is, 'I was hungry, and I didn't bring any good food with me, and I madly decided I would rather eat anything than stay hungry.'

3. **State what you intend to do next time.**

   'Tomorrow I will bring a healthy snack to work with me.'

Chapter 10

Navigating Eating Out and Special Occasions

In This Chapter

▶ Adopting strategies for eating out successfully

▶ Staying on track while eating in social situations

▶ Minding your sugar intake during vacations, holidays and special occasions

*O*nce you get your day-to-day eating under control at home and at work, eating well when you're out at restaurants or celebrating special occasions begins to get easier. While restaurants often have tempting dishes that aren't so healthy for us, most are also smart enough to have healthy options. Even McDonald's and KFC are trying to go down that path. You just have to be brave and ask for what you want. The restaurant industry can't afford to sit back and not adjust their menu to the expanding climate of health and wellness. In addition to asking at restaurants, you can ask or seek out what you want and need at dinner parties, birthdays or other celebrations. This is all very manageable, and our clients have been trying it for years.

In this chapter, we give you strategies for making smart choices at restaurants and tips for eating out without making yourself feel like you have a food hangover the next day. We also discuss ways for you to eat reasonably during the holidays and other special events, so you can still enjoy yourself while sticking to your low-sugar goals.

Eating Out Joyfully

Mindfulness and planning are very important to prevent the act of eating out from turning into a nutritional disaster. Some restaurants may serve up enticing entrees and mains topped with sauces loaded with trans fat and hidden sugar, and often they deliver portions that are double the size of your 'norm'. Dessert menus may break the 'sugar-celibacy' and move into 'carbicide'. However, the key to staying in control is to remember you are in the driver's seat of your decisions.

Watching portion sizes

When eating out at a restaurant, it's common to be served more than you would normally eat at home (depending on the kind of restaurant). Here are some tips to stay in control:

- ✔ **Pay attention to how much you eat, how fast you eat, and whether you really need any more food in your stomach.** Refer to Chapter 8 for more advice on mindfulness and proactive eating.

- ✔ **Eat vegetables first, then protein.** After that, decide whether you really want (or need) any of the extra carbs or starches (such as rice, pasta and bread) on your plate.

- ✔ **Ask the wait staff to put what you don't eat in a takeaway container (if possible).** This request is quite common in America, and is becoming more common in Australia and New Zealand. Most restaurants feel privileged that you have enjoyed the food enough to take it home for a second meal.

Making room for alcohol and dessert

If you don't eat out very often, it's okay to make the experience special. Don't put yourself in food jail on your birthday or anniversary — go ahead and indulge in something that you ordinarily wouldn't eat. Just don't go so far overboard that you create a 'food baby' in your stomach and regret it later. When you eat out for a special occasion, have some wine, a white spirit with soda water and lime (not a sweet mixed drink like a cosmopolitan or a mojito) or a beer, and choose between an entree and a dessert with your main, but not both. And for the record, you're not required to eat all of whatever you choose!

If you eat out several times per week, the restaurant experience is no longer special; it's just a method of feeding yourself. Treat your day-to-day restaurant meals just like you would any other — minding your sugar content, portions, protein/carb ratios, and other standard nutrition variables that you've learned to pay attention to. Ask for an extra salad or extra green vegetables instead of chips or potatoes. Truly, it is quite okay to ask. Don't get caught up in the moment and not register what you're eating — *what* you eat is much more important than *where* you eat it.

Staying mindful

When you're eating out at a restaurant or at a party, chances are that everyone's focus is on the conversation and company instead of the food, so be careful not to use external cues (like an empty plate) as the only signals for when you've had enough to eat. Frequently turn your attention inward and pay attention to what you're doing and how you're feeling. Ask yourself questions like

- ✔ Am I eating too fast or not chewing thoroughly?
- ✔ Do I really need more food or could I stop eating right now?
- ✔ How does my stomach feel?
- ✔ How much have I had to drink?
- ✔ When was the last time I really tasted what I was eating?

When looking over the menu, be sure that all the basic nutrition bases are covered in your decisions: Double-check that you have vegetables and protein on your plate, that your choice is low-sugar, and that your portions are reasonable. Smart decisions when ordering make it easier to temper your behaviour while eating. Refer to Chapter 5 for an overview of nutrition basics.

Choosing the basics

If you're worried about sugar content, kilojoules or other dietary considerations when eating out (and you should at least be thinking about these), you can't go wrong with vegetables and lean protein. Endless varieties of delicious meals are available that are heavy on veggies and protein and low on sugar, starches and sauces. When in doubt, your best bet basics are meals with a protein source (chicken, fish, lamb, beef and so on) and a pile of vegetables without too much stuff on them. Often, an organic mixed green salad topped with salmon, prawns or chicken tossed in a simple vinaigrette can be one of the most delightful dishes on the menu, not to mention a healthy alternative to some of the many kilojoule- and sugar-laden main courses available.

If you're not sure how something on the menu is prepared, don't be afraid to ask. Most kitchens are happy to make you a version of a dish without the sauce or to come up with a simple alternative. Having worked in restaurant kitchens ourselves (and Michele even owns a restaurant), we can say that sometimes it's a nice change for the chef to come up with a healthier alternative.

Navigating Social Eating

Staying on track while eating in social situations — dinner parties, date nights, wedding receptions and similar events — can be challenging. But, once you understand how to make it work, you will be so thankful the following day. Typically, the fare served by caterers and restaurants is higher in sugar, fat, kilojoules and portion size than what you'd ordinarily eat, and you'll likely be focused on everything except what (and how) you're eating. Being aware of your food intake while fully participating in all the social interaction takes some practice, but by utilising a few of the basic skills in the following sections, you should be able to stay proactive with your food and still have a great time!

Preventing common mistakes

If you can avoid these common pitfalls, you'll have a much easier time keeping the event from turning into an eating disaster:

- ✔ **Eating everything you're given:** Many events have a constant flow of food coming at you from all directions, much of it carbohydrates. News flash — you don't have to eat everything that someone hands you. Choose your snacks wisely. Michele's former clients use the phrase 'choose your poison' — meaning, for example, are you going to have a glass of wine? If the answer is 'Yes', don't also have the high-carb meat pie that's coming around. Go for the crust-less quiche or the chicken skewer — both of which hardly have any sugar — because you know you will be getting some sugar in the wine.

- ✔ **Playing the 'I'll have some if you have some' game:** People often look toward another's behaviour to give them permission to eat dessert or junk food. Just because your friend wants some dessert doesn't mean you're obligated to eat some too. It's not rude for one person not to eat something that others are eating, so don't fall into the social trap of using what others do as an excuse not to make your own decisions. Also watch out for the 'frenemy' — the friend who is really an enemy and is a little bit jealous that you're reaping the benefits of a low-sugar way of life, such as good skin, balanced moods, weight loss, vibrancy and a positive, controlled outlook on life.

- ✔ **Staying near the food all night:** People love to congregate in the kitchen or near the food, but conversations don't have to stay there all night. You can be the one who invites people to move to a different area by saying something like, 'Let's move away from these pies before I eat them all.' You may even be helping out some others who may be trying to organise their eating too. If you stand and talk next to the desserts plate all night, you're just asking for trouble!

Being prepared

If you're headed to a place or an event where you know that the food will be unhealthy, plan ahead and arrive having already eaten a healthy, sugar-free meal. If you arrive hungry and all that's available is junk food, you'll probably succumb to your hunger and unravel all the good planning you've worked hard on.

If you're not able to eat a full, healthy meal before a social dining event, at least make sure that you eat often enough throughout the day so you don't arrive ravenous. Walking into a room filled with tempting finger food when you haven't eaten for six or seven hours is a disaster waiting to happen. Plan ahead!

Creating balance

As discussed in Chapter 8, beware of becoming obsessive or neurotic about food. If you're at a special event and you spend all your time and energy being super-strict about what you eat, you may find that you feel disappointed even though you ate well.

We've heard clients talk about an event or party with fear in their voices, simply because they knew desserts would be there. If you have that attitude, you'll most likely have a miserable time no matter what the event because you'll be so afraid you may succumb to the allure of sugar that you won't be able to relax and enjoy yourself. This is both sad and unhealthy. Empower yourself, and always remember that you're the one who makes every single decision about your actions and your attitude.

One of the keys to creating balance with eating is that you must feel good about doing it. If having desserts and treats in moderation feels like punishment, you'll feel like it's dieting instead of normal eating, and you won't be likely to maintain the moderate approach for long. Refer to Chapter 9 for tips on the important concept of creating a 'new normal'.

We encourage you to allow yourself to eat a reasonable amount of junk food at a special event. Just do it with purpose, not unconsciously, and stay mindful about what you choose to do — no 'brain off' gluttony allowed! Limit your portions of sugar-laden food to a few bites, and eat slowly. If you find that you're not enjoying what you're eating, don't finish it.

Reprogramming an all-or-nothing attitude about sweets

An all-or-nothing attitude toward food is one of the most dangerous traps for the sugar addict. If you try to remain on an overly restrictive eating plan, you'll eventually give in to your cravings because hardly anyone can stay on an 'absolutely none' plan for very long. When you give in to your old habits, the all-or-nothing mindset will swing you to the other end of the spectrum, and you'll overindulge and get caught back on the sugar roller-coaster.

The problem with having an all-or-nothing mentality is that you treat your improved eating plan as a temporary restriction, not as a new way of eating or thinking about food. Reprogramming the all-or-nothing attitude allows you to enjoy all foods in your diet, even some dessert, just not with complete abandon. Your goal with improved eating habits should be to create a 'new normal' so that you never feel like you're on a diet or a restricted eating plan (refer to Chapter 9).

A party, an event or a holiday is *not* the last time you'll have the opportunity to eat your favourite treats. When you have a new normal, you don't follow a strict diet, so you aren't deprived of these foods forever. When you decide to indulge in a treat, have a few bites, and then say 'enough'. You don't have to eat a lifetime of sugar in one night!

Surviving Vacations and Special Occasions

Throughout the course of a year, you're likely to experience stretches of time where sugar and junk food are plentiful, like vacations and holidays. The tips in the following sections can help you keep tabs on your sugar intake while still enjoying some treats in moderation during these times. These tips guide you through making the best choices out of whatever food is available to help you stay on track. Too many people come home from their holidays feeling bloated and puffy, and with digestive problems; that isn't a holiday.

Vacations

When you're on vacation, throwing moderation to the wind is easy, especially if you're in a situation where high-sugar food is omnipresent. Cutting loose and lightening up on what you allow yourself to eat while on vacation is okay, but if you pull out all the stops and go overboard, you can do a lot of damage in a short period of time.

Vacation should be a time for you to relax, get out of your normal routine, spend some quality time with family or friends, and soak up some special life experiences. Some indulgent cuisine can be part of that, but the focus of your vacation shouldn't be stuffing yourself with as many carbohydrates as you can find. Keep your focus on decompressing and on enjoying great experiences, not on seeing how much you can devour from the dessert bar before you make yourself sick. You should not need a vacation from food when you return from your vacation.

Holidays and the festive season

Have you noticed how many people completely shut off any sensibility or moderation around food during holidays such as Christmas? When they give themselves permission to indulge in some holiday sweets, an all-or-nothing mentality takes over, and they go completely overboard, gobbling down every single sugar-filled treat they can lay their hands on — usually with the promise that at the beginning of the new year they'll start their diet, get back to the gym or whatever other promise they make to themselves every year. It's almost like they've entered a contest in their mind, trying to win the award for who can cram the most sugar in before January. Michele likes to refer to the after-effects of this approach as 'Christmas-itis' — that is, the ill feeling you get from all that holiday cheer.

During holidays, you don't need to splurge at every meal of every day. The holiday season isn't a pass to eat foolishly for weeks! Do some planning in advance and look for times when it will be easy for you to put together a healthy meal. Be on the lookout for situations in which you'll want to overindulge, and be judicious about which ones you allow to become major deviations from your healthy, low-sugar lifestyle. Choose your food battles and make conscious, sensible decisions about when you have a treat and how much of it you eat.

During the festive season, don't lose sight of the big picture of a healthy nutrition plan — that is, the importance of things like vegetables, protein, water and portion control. Consider junk food as extra, not as a substitute for real food. Be sure to portion out your treat before you start eating so you can keep the amount of sugar you consume in check. You don't have to eat *all* the biscuits to enjoy them!

Birthdays and other special occasions

Just because you're celebrating a special occasion, such as a birthday or an anniversary, doesn't mean you must eat foolishly. Don't feel obligated to eat dessert or drink too much to get the most out of your celebration. Focus on the special people around you instead of the junk food that's available.

Past conditioning may have led you to believe that it's okay to eat all bad foods on special occasions. This unhealthy mindset reinforces sugar as a reward or as a necessary part of special times.

A good strategy to help you stay on your low-sugar lifestyle during special occasions is to distinguish between healthy hunger and a food frenzy. *Healthy hunger* is when you want to eat because you listen to the cues that your body gives you, and you're actually hungry. *Food frenzy* is when you want to eat because you see something that looks enticing. Stay mindful by paying attention to what your body tells you, and don't allow your eyes to dictate your mouth's behaviour. The next time you get a craving to eat something, pause for a moment to assess whether you're truly healthy hungry or mentally walking into a food frenzy.

Chapter 11

Getting a Boost from Your Support System

· ·

In This Chapter

▶ Dealing with other people's negativity

▶ Building a support system among family, friends and co-workers

▶ Using support groups and internet forums to stay on track

▶ Getting professional help

· ·

*A*s you begin your quest to beat sugar addiction and lead a healthier lifestyle, building a support system around you encourages you and helps hold you accountable. A support system also gives you a close ring of people with whom you can share both your triumphs and your setbacks.

In this chapter, we share some ideas for building a reliable support system — who to include, who not to include and how to be prepared for the saboteurs you may encounter. We give you some tips for bringing your family on board and lay out some options for support groups that you may not have thought of. Lastly, we present some advice for choosing the right professional help when you need it.

Building Your 'Feel Good' Resilience

When it comes to food, not following the herd can be challenging. If you announce to your friends and family that you've decided to overcome your addiction to sugar, be prepared for some unexpected reactions. Though some people will congratulate you and wish you the best, others will react as if you're declaring war on them and on their own favourite foods. Be prepared for people who you thought were your friends to make snide remarks, to tell you you're crazy, or to waffle on about how you'll never be able to sustain the low-sugar lifestyle. Do your best to ignore these people. Gaining approval from every person you know isn't important. Every day, as you continue to feel good about yourself, you'll become more resilient to what others may say.

When you're met with scepticism, don't fall victim to other people's fears and negativity. Keep in mind that you're not completely banning sugar from your life; you're just changing the way you usually do things and making better decisions about your physical body, mental clarity and overall vitality.

Eating better isn't a battle; in fact, when you get control of your eating, it's joyous. That sounds strange but you get a lot of pride and joy from owning your health, eating well and feeling good about yourself. Taking better care of yourself is merely a series of ongoing smart decisions that lead you where you want to go, both physically and emotionally. Focus on consistency, not on waging war against food. Consult Chapter 9 for tips on creating a new, healthy 'normal'.

Bringing Your Family On Board

By trying to get your family to cooperate in your endeavours to eat better, you may end up with a loving circle of family support or you may end up completely disappointed. What's often important is getting yourself in a healthy, balanced place before you even consider helping others.

As your enthusiasm, your mood, your skin and your physical body begin to shine from your low-sugar transformation, you'll feel excited and you're likely going to want to take everyone you know on this ride. Just remember that you can't change other people; you can only change yourself!

Families off Sugar — the FOS program

The health risks associated with childhood obesity are regularly discussed, but kids' emotional risks are sometimes forgotten. Overweight children are often teased at school, in the playground, and even at home. They suffer physically inside and out, but they severely suffer emotionally with lack of self-esteem. They look different from other children and know it, but they can't make the changes they need to make on their own. As an adult, you can take on this shift on your own, but children need adult help to shop, support and guide.

The vicious cycle of being overweight or obese as a result of diet is the same vicious cycle that some teenage patients get into when dealing with anxiety, depression or attention deficit hyperactivity disorder (ADHD). Nutrition is not always the root cause of anxiety, depression, ADHD, hormonal imbalances or skin conditions (what Michele refers to as 'self-esteem bombs'), but with a whole-food, low-sugar diet, these health issues are improved dramatically.

A Healthy View has instituted Families off Sugar (FOS), a program that aims to help combat the epidemic of childhood obesity and sugar self-esteem bombs that teenagers are facing. The team of nutritionists in this program work with a GP, family counsellors and exercise specialists, with the goal of helping the entire family change its lifestyle.

A family approach is the best route if a child in the family is battling with self-esteem bombs due to poor nutritional choices. If the parents are on board with a healthy lifestyle, the pantry and refrigerator are often stocked appropriately too. Aside from the FOS program, many nutritionists are available who have a whole-food approach and don't put families on restrictive diets or ban all treats. Losing weight and gaining mental clarity shouldn't be a punishment. Every child or teen is different but generally a nutritional program should include adjustments to the family's diet, implement regular exercise, and teach the family how to plan a weekly menu and buy healthy foods within their financial budget.

Even without the help of professionals to advise and assist, you can apply the following tenets to your own family's routine to reap health benefits:

5   Eat *five* servings of fruits and vegetables each day. Include two fruit and at least three vegetables.

4   Eat together as a family at least *four* times a week. Your shared meal doesn't always have to be dinner but you need to connect at a meal at least four times through the week.

3   Eat *three* healthy meals a day — no skipping meals, especially breakfast.

2   Limit screen time (computer, TV, Facebook and video games) to less than *two* hours a day.

1   Aim for *one* session of physical activity each day. (A session is 30 to 60 minutes.)

0   Reduce the number of sugar-sweetened drinks like soft drinks, flavoured milk and juice to *zero*.

Try gradually implementing these changes into your family's lifestyle, and watch your waistlines shrink and everyone's self-esteem and health skyrocket.

Consult Chapter 9 for tips on gradually introducing healthier foods into your household.

Enlisting Friends, Family and Co-Workers

Confiding in a small group of friends, family or co-workers who know you can strengthen your support system. However, involving the right friends is important because you may not receive the right kind of support from everyone you know. The following sections explain how to involve the right people and how to avoid those who will drag you down.

Supporters

The ideal support partners are friends who truly support your goals to free yourself from the grip of sugar. They may have seen your struggle with your weight, concentration, mood or energy levels, or any of the sugar-laden conditions. Tell them that you really want and need a healthier life that's under control. Confide in them that you're telling them because you need their gentle support, not because you're asking them to come with you on this low-sugar journey; you simply want their encouragement and understanding about this change in your life.

You'll probably receive the best support and accountability from friends who are looking to improve their own eating habits and lifestyles, even if they're not your closest friends. Your best ally may turn out to be someone you barely know! Look for people in your circle who are already living the lifestyle you aspire to. You may even find yourself doing things with these supporters that you never would have considered before — for example, yoga, bush walks, meditation classes or jogging. You may find this slow transition off sugar will lead to new hobbies.

Saboteurs

Regardless of how close you feel to your friends and family members, we guarantee that some of them will unknowingly act as saboteurs, so be emotionally resilient and ready for this to happen. You'll have friends or co-workers who may make fun of you for your food choices at restaurants, or your spouse may bring home an ice-cream cake the day after you have a tearful conversation about how out of control you feel your life is.

Try to keep in mind that these people are (hopefully) not being mean or insensitive on purpose; they just don't understand how hard making life changes can be. They probably haven't considered making any improvements for themselves or just don't understand what you're going through because they've never tried to overcome any type of addiction.

Whatever the reason for their behaviour, try not to hold it against them. People who aren't interested in adopting healthy behaviours themselves often engage in negative talk about yours or downplay the importance of the changes you're trying to make. Sometimes, they're quietly envious of your new vibrancy and sense of purpose. Breaking an addiction and moving forward takes a very strong person. Be proud and don't let other people discourage you!

Don't bother talking about nutritional or low-sugar stuff or exercise with saboteurs — they're just not interested and they'll only bring you down. You may leave the conversation with self-doubt, so just switch topics immediately. You have plenty of other things to talk about, so reserve discussions about your personal goals and progress for supportive people who are interested in hearing about your journey.

If you have a friend with whom you often share 'naughty' treats (such as dessert, wine or cocktails) don't be surprised if they try to tempt you. Don't let a distorted sense of loyalty dictate your behaviour! Your friend doesn't need you to eat junk food to enjoy your time together, and you haven't abandoned your friend if you decide not to partake in sugary treats that the two of you have historically shared. Be resilient and smile and feel good inside. End of story!

Finding a Support Group

Collaborating with other people with similar goals and experiences can be a helpful way to share pitfalls and celebrations, especially if they're in similar circumstances. Sometimes, staying on track is easier if you're part of a team in which everyone has the same goal. Hearing others' stories can help validate your own experiences, and sharing your own experiences and advice can help others. Michele has had a number of clients who have come to her for one-on-one consultations. These clients have then joined a cleanse retreat or a 'cleanse at home' group and, surprisingly, the group situation was far more effective. When asking the 'cleansers' why their nutritional achievements differed in the different environments, they responded that, while they felt educated and supported with both of the programs, being encouraged by their small group made them part of a team that had similar issues to conquer.

Getting involved with a local support group

Getting involved in a group therapy session can be an easy way to build a team of support around you. Support groups for various eating issues abound, or you could even start your own! Here are some tips for finding a group to visit:

- ✓ Ask a GP, a therapist or counsellor to recommend a local nutritionist or support group that's appropriate for you.

- ✓ Peruse church community bulletin boards for notifications of group meetings.

- ✓ Contact the National Eating Disorders Collaboration (NEDC; www.nedc.com.au) for group support.

If you or someone you know is struggling with an eating disorder or negative body image, contact The Butterfly Foundation (www. thebutterflyfoundation.org.au) or the Australia & New Zealand Academy for Eating Disorders (anzaed.org.au).

Investigating internet forums

Internet discussion groups are another option for finding advice and motivation. Peers and professionals from all over the world can share stories, struggles and advice. Internet forums can be great places to obtain general support and encouragement, especially if you're struggling with setbacks. They also afford you a wonderful opportunity to give back to the community by being there for others when they need the same.

Unfortunately, internet forums have a downside too. The anonymous nature of the internet makes it easy for people to post incorrect, angry or downright offensive comments on group discussion boards. You may also run into evangelists of particular diets or products who are critical of all other diets and products, so be prepared to weed through a lot of negative postings. You'll also encounter a lot of salespeople for particular products. Again, be resilient.

Seeking Help from a Professional

Overhauling a lifetime of destructive food habits can be a daunting task, especially when you also have a lot of other issues with work and family on your plate. Finding a professional therapist or counsellor who has helped hundreds of people in your shoes is a smart way to propel your personal growth to a new level, especially if you're struggling with some deep emotional issues like depression, self-criticism or hopelessness.

One of the things we consistently hear from clients is, 'I know what to do; I just can't seem to do it.' Because doing is indeed much harder than knowing, receiving some guidance from a professional can help you develop some strategies and tricks to implement the healthy changes that you're having difficulty making on your own.

Nutrition counsellors

If you have a challenging health condition like type 2 diabetes, metabolic syndrome, insulin issues, polycystic ovarian syndrome (PCOS), digestive issues, kidney disease, thyroid dysfunction, cognitive issues or food allergies, we suggest that you find a qualified nutritionist who has experience with that particular condition to assist you with your dietary journey. Contact the Australian Traditional Medical Society (www.atms.com.au) for a qualified nutritionist.

Food coaches aren't the same as nutritionists. Food coaches can offer great advice on general food and health topics, but don't have experience with specific health conditions — for advice on these conditions, seek out practitioners with a degree or advanced diploma in nutrition. It's also best to check that a practitioner belongs to an accredited governing body.

During your first nutrition appointment, if your practitioner hands you a photocopy of the food pyramid or stares blankly at you when you mention probiotic supplements or whey protein, find a different health professional who's more educated in current evidence-based nutrition science.

Consider asking your chiropractor, massage therapist, and/or fitness trainer to recommend a qualified, well-rounded nutrition counsellor with whom their clients have had good success.

Therapists

A trained professional such as a therapist or psychologist can help you delve into the hows and whys of your behaviour, emotions and beliefs. Finding an experienced therapist to help guide you through the introspection process is time and money well spent!

Finding a therapist who's a good fit for you may take some time and experimentation. This field has many different approaches and personalities, so be prepared to try out several practitioners until you find one who feels right.

Check with your local professional body to find a psychologist in your area. In Australia, check www.psychology.org.au/findapsychologist, or go to www.buddhismandpsychotherapy.org for mindfulness-trained Buddhist counsellors and therapists. In New Zealand, check www.psychology.org.nz/Find_a_Psychologist.

Finding a professional who's good is much more important than finding one who's convenient. Selecting a therapist just because his office is on your way home probably won't yield the best match for you. Doing your own personal work is important, life-changing stuff, so treat it accordingly!

Before booking your first session, talk to the therapist or the receptionist on the phone and get answers to questions like:

- How many years have you been in this industry and what are your credentials?
- What are your areas of expertise?
- Do you have experience with issues like mine?

While you're on the phone, ask about payment, cancellation policies and health-care rebates.

Chapter 12

Sugar-Busting Moves: Incorporating Exercise

- -

In This Chapter

▶ Understanding the relationship between sugar and metabolism

▶ Following a consistent, manageable exercise schedule

▶ Designing cardiovascular and strength training exercise programs

▶ Doing strength training exercises correctly

▶ Starting out with some example workouts

- -

*P*eople often report a lifetime of frustration with exercise. Even if you can find the time, motivation and energy to make exercise a regular part of your week, it's easy to get confused by all the conflicting exercise advice that gets thrown at you from magazines, exercise evangelists, misinformed-but-well-intentioned bloggers and TV gurus.

Adequate and appropriate exercise is a vital component of long-term health, and it's especially important for the sugar addict who wants to lose weight and stay craving-free. In this chapter, Dan takes you through the effects a proper exercise program can have on your body and lays out the key elements for constructing a successful exercise plan.

Instead of making promises to yourself to start hitting the treadmill yet again, we urge you to take the time to read through this chapter in detail so you can understand the kind of workouts that you need to do. Dan explains the effectiveness and the proper structure of basic strength training and cardiovascular workouts, so you'll have an efficient, effective system of exercise to help you slim down, get in shape and stay away from sugar.

Getting a medical check-up before beginning any exercise program is prudent. A screening by your GP can uncover a hidden problem like a heart defect, a tumour or arterial blockage that needs to be addressed before you undertake any change in physical activity.

Seeing How Exercise Affects Sugar Metabolism

Some of the worst effects of a high-sugar diet are fat storage and insulin resistance (refer to Chapter 4). The good news is that regular exercise can reverse both of those!

Exercise improves insulin sensitivity and your cholesterol profile. Improved function of the insulin receptors means that your body produces less insulin and stores less fat. Along with higher protein and vegetable intake and reduced simple carbohydrate intake, regular exercise is the most important treatment for type 2 diabetes.

Strength training is an important part of losing weight because lifting weights increases your metabolism so you burn more kilojoules doing everything, even sitting down reading this book (stand up and keep reading!). Exercise burns up your muscles' stores of carbohydrate (called *muscle glycogen*), so when you eat carbohydrates after you work out, your body uses the carbs to refuel your muscles instead of storing them as fat. Exercise also suppresses *ghrelin* (the hunger hormone), thus decreasing your appetite and limiting cravings.

In addition to these beneficial effects on sugar metabolism, exercise reduces stress, improves brain function, reduces arthritis pain, elevates mood, improves the immune system, increases flexibility and strengthens bones! If you can get your exercise outdoors and in the sunshine (in the morning or afternoon), you're getting a double bang for your buck, because you're getting all the benefits we just mentioned plus an increase in your vitamin D supply.

Sticking to an Exercise Schedule

The biggest obstacle to regular exercise is finding the time to do it. Everyone is busy, and most people overbook their schedules to the point that they don't have any time for self-care. To be healthy, this must change! Exercise doesn't take a lot of time, but you do have to be consistent to have success, which means you have to put workouts on your schedule, just like you do any other important commitment. New research shows that for optimum weight management you should exercise above 150 minutes per week, which is at least five 30-minute blocks of exercise each week. Finding this time shouldn't be too difficult. (Funny that most people can easily find time for 90 minutes of television each week but complain that they can't find this same time for exercise.)

Setting realistic goals is an important component of success. If you tell yourself you're going to work out every day (and you don't have to, by the way), you'll either stress yourself out trying to commit that much time or feel like a failure and quit as soon as you miss a few days. Set a realistic goal of three half-hour blocks each week and put them on your calendar.

Your 30 minutes of exercise don't have to happen all at once. Studies show that three 10-minute bouts of exercise yield the same health improvements as one 30-minute session. The metabolic effects of just 10 minutes of exercise last at least an hour!

Reaping the Benefits of Being Consistent

Consistency is one of the most important parts of making an exercise program work for you. We live in a cause-and-effect universe, so you can't expect any improvements if you don't put in the time and effort to get them.

Exercise programming is based on the concept of *progressive overload* — taxing the body just a little bit more than it considers normal so that it's forced to adapt to the new demands that are imposed on it. That's how your body gradually gets stronger, healthier and in better physical condition. Here are some benefits you can expect to gain from your continued progress:

- ✔ Activities of daily life improve with higher levels of fitness.
- ✔ Balance, quick reactions, and *proprioception* (body awareness) are strong deterrents to injury.
- ✔ Bone density improvements are markedly better with heavier weights and athletic moves like jumping.
- ✔ Fit people burn more fat when they exercise than unfit people.
- ✔ High levels of fitness improve your immune system.
- ✔ Higher levels of fitness open the door to more exercise options, thus avoiding boredom and burnout.
- ✔ It feels really good to be able to run a charity race with your kids and keep up.
- ✔ Building muscle content has more anti-ageing impact than stress or genetics.
- ✔ You burn more kilojoules with a higher-intensity exercise session.
- ✔ You experience more health benefits with higher levels of fitness.
- ✔ Your skin receives more nutrients with exercise due to better blood flow.

Comparing Exercise Types

The exercise physiology field separates exercise into two major categories: *cardiovascular* exercise (also known as *cardio* or *aerobic exercise*) and *strength training* (also called *resistance training* or *weight training*).

Cardiovascular exercise

Cardio (aerobic) exercise involves repetitive body movements that can be sustained for long periods (for many minutes or, in cases like a marathon or the Tour de France, even hours). Cardiovascular exercise uses your body's *aerobic system* of energy, which means that it uses oxygen, stored carbohydrate, body fat and a small amount of protein for fuel. Examples of cardio exercise are walking, jogging, cycling, jumping rope, swimming laps and using the stair climbers or elliptical gizmos at the gym.

Cardio exercise improves the condition of your *cardiorespiratory system* (heart, lungs and circulatory system), burns kilojoules, and improves glucose metabolism and insulin sensitivity.

Strength training exercise

Strength training uses an external resistance against your muscles' contractions during certain types of movements. The resistance can come from weights, exercise tubing, body weight, or any number of fun and exotic things like sandbags, medicine balls and kettlebells. The key factor of strength training is that the resistance must be great enough to make the muscles tire after a relatively small number of contractions (typically 8 to 12 repetitions).

Strength training yields the same health benefits as cardiovascular exercise, and many additional benefits. Both burn similar numbers of kilojoules (300 to 500 kilojoules per typical session), but strength training is superior for a number of reasons:

- ✓ Strength training delivers all the health benefits of cardiovascular exercise, plus the additional benefits of increased strength, improved bone density, better flexibility, increased metabolic boost, and postural and cosmetic improvements (healthy skin).

- ✓ Strength training results in higher *post-exercise oxygen consumption* rates (and longer durations) than cardio, meaning you burn more kilojoules after your workout.

- ✓ Strength training develops your muscles, which elevates your metabolism, so you burn more kilojoules doing everything all day!

Combining cardio and strength training

If you're pressed for time and have to pick either strength training or cardiovascular exercise, you should select strength training because you get so much more bang for your time and effort. If you have time to do both, do your workout in this order:

1. **Warm up with some gentle cardio and a few stretches.**

2. **Do your strength training workout.**

3. **Do your cardio exercise.**

4. **Cool down and stretch.** If you need some stretching guidance, see the instructional videos at `http://au.dummies.com/how-to/content/the-rules-of-stretching.html`.

5. **Eat a protein and carbohydrate combination within 45 minutes of finishing your workout.**

To lose one kilogram of body fat per week, you need to burn an additional 37,000 kilojoules per week, or around 5,000 kilojoules (about 1,200 calories) per day.

Staying motivated

If you're not in great shape when you start off, staying on track with your exercise program can be a challenge. If you're a beginner, exercise isn't yet a lifestyle habit for you, so it's still something you have to plan for and put on your schedule. Your workouts may feel underwhelming or you may feel embarrassed or ashamed of how hard it is for you or how quickly you tire out. Stick with it! It gets better. Here are a few tips to help keep your motivation high:

✔ Get a friend to join the exercise program with you. Having a buddy to help you stay on track never hurts.

✔ Chart your achievements so you can see a visual representation of your progress.

✔ Share your successes with friends and family. They will be proud of you.

✔ Read other people's success stories on blogs or support group websites (refer to Chapter 11). If they can do it, so can you!

Something else that may help motivate you: High-intensity workouts burn more kilojoules than low-intensity workouts, and therefore take less time. As you get in better shape, you'll be able to work harder, so you can look forward to shorter workouts!

Fit individuals burn a greater percentage of fat for energy — 70 per cent at rest versus less than 50 per cent for those who are unfit. Fit people also mobilise their fat stores sooner compared to unfit people. The more consistent you are with your workout plan, the better shape you get in, and the more effective your workouts get!

Creating a Cardiovascular Exercise Program

Cardiovascular exercise is the simplest kind of exercise. If you walk, jog, dance or hike, you don't need any special equipment, and you can exercise pretty much anywhere and at any time. Cardio exercise generally requires no practice or special skills, and it provides an easy way to work up a good sweat, burn some extra kilojoules, loosen your stiff muscles and clear your head.

Don't fall into the trap of spending a majority of your exercise time doing only cardio work. Cardio burns kilojoules, improves your insulin sensitivity and gets your circulatory system in better shape — all good things. But a high-intensity strength circuit (see the section 'Developing a Strength Training Workout' later in the chapter) does all that, plus it raises your metabolism, increases your strength and bone density, improves your posture, tones your muscles, burns fat, and improves your core stability and balance. Put most of your time and effort into your weight training workouts, and do cardio as an extra.

Choosing your cardio activity

So many clients ask, 'Which cardio exercise (or cardio machine) should I use?' Basically, they're all the same.

The purpose of cardiovascular exercise is to elevate your heart rate and respiration for a particular length of time. Cardio doesn't tax your muscles enough to stimulate much muscular development, so asking which cardio gizmo works your legs more (or hips or butt or whatever body part you're trying to target) is moot. Your *level of exertion* — how high your heart rate gets and how hard you breathe — determines how many kilojoules you burn. Whether you're jogging, cycling, using the elliptical machine, jumping rope or swimming, the benefits are determined by how hard you exercise, not by the kind of cardio you pick.

The best cardio to choose is one you enjoy — or at least one you don't hate. You have hundreds of ways to exercise, so pick something you don't dread. Mix it up so you don't get bored and maybe pop some headphones on to enjoy your favourite music. Joining a group fitness class can also help with the boredom factor and add a more social element to your exercise.

Determining duration and frequency

At the time of writing, these are the physical activity guidelines for adults from the Australian Department of Health and Ageing:

- ✔ **Incorporate activity into your daily life as much as you can.** Walk or cycle instead of using the car, and think of moving your body as an opportunity, rather than an inconvenience.

- ✔ **Add at least 30 minutes moderate-intensity physical activity to your routine on most (preferably all) days.** These 30 minutes can be broken up through the day.

- ✔ **If possible, also add some regular, vigorous activity.** This is in addition to (rather than instead of) the two preceding points, and can help you achieve greater health and fitness.

For more information on these guidelines (including physical activity guidelines for children) see http://www.health.gov.au/internet/main/publishing.nsf/Content/health-pubhlth-strateg-phys-act-guidelines.

Any exercise is better than none! If you're unable to meet these minimums, you can still benefit from some activity. Do *something!*

Squeezing in extra activity

Sitting for long periods of time *(sedentary behaviour)* has been shown to be a health risk all by itself, independent of exercise habits. Meeting the guidelines for physical activity doesn't negate the health risks that come from sitting all day. Time spent watching TV or working on a computer adds up and increases health risks over time. Get up and move as often as you can!

Here are some ways you can break up the monotony of sitting and increase your daily activity level without blocking out any more time:

- ✔ If you have a desk job, stand up and walk around or do a few stretches every 30 or 60 minutes.

- ✔ March in place while you watch TV or brush your teeth.

- ✔ Stand up (and pace or stand on one leg if you feel like it) while you're on the phone or reading. Some companies encourage standing during meetings instead of sitting.

- ✔ Take the stairs instead of the lift or escalator.

- ✔ When you get out of the car, walk one lap around the parking lot before you go inside (unless you're going into the gym).

Finding the right difficulty level

The difficulty or intensity of cardiovascular exercise is determined by how high your heart rate gets. When gauging the intensity of your cardio exercise, you can either assess how hard you feel like you're working (self-perception) or get more precise and measure your actual pulse rate.

If you'd like to keep things simple, use a scale of 1 to 10 during your cardio exercise to describe how hard you feel like you're working:

1 = Am I lying in a hammock or am I exercising?

3 = I'm doing something but it's very, very easy.

5 = This isn't too hard; I could do this for at least an hour. (Activities in this category may include walking, hiking or working in the garden, for example.)

7 = I'm working pretty hard; I'll tire out relatively soon.

10 = I'm exerting the absolute maximum effort I can before I pass out or my heart explodes.

Here's how to determine your pulse rate: Using your index and middle fingers, find your pulse, either on your neck next to your windpipe or on your wrist straight down from your index finger. Count the beats for 10 seconds, and then multiply that number by 6 to get your *beats per minute* (bpm).

While you're at rest, your normal heart rate should range from the low 50s to about 85 bpm. In general, the better condition you're in, the lower your resting heart rate is because your heart and vascular system are more efficient.

You can make it your goal to keep your heart rate elevated to a specific target number, known as your *target heart rate*, and keep it there for a predetermined amount of time. While doing your cardiovascular exercise, check your pulse rate periodically to determine whether you're working at your target heart rate. If your heart rate is below your target range, pick up the pace. If it's too high, slow down so you can stay in your target range.

To determine your target heart rate, you must first calculate your predicted maximum heart rate, which is 208 minus 70 per cent of your age. That's the estimated maximum speed your heart can beat. For example, if you're 46 years old, your predicted maximum heart rate is 176 beats per minute: 70 per cent of 46 is 32; 208 − 32 = 176. You don't need to exercise at your absolute maximum effort, so you find your target heart rate by taking a percentage of your predicted maximum:

- 50 to 60 per cent if you're very out of shape or on heart medication

- 70 to 85 per cent for general fitness conditioning ('getting in shape')

- 90 to 100 per cent for high-intensity intervals or sport-specific athletic training

Using the example of a 46 year old, the target heart rate ranges (in beats per minute) would be:

- 88 to 106 bpm (50 to 60 per cent of 176) for those who are very out of shape or on heart medication

- 123 to 150 bpm (70 to 85 per cent of 176) for general fitness conditioning

- 158 to 176 bpm (90 to 100 per cent of 176) for high-intensity intervals or sport-specific athletic training

Certain medical conditions or prescription medications can artificially suppress your heart rate. If you have any medical conditions or take medication that affects your heart rate (medications for blood pressure, most commonly), you should get some professional help to set up a safe and appropriate exercise program (see the sidebar 'Finding a fitness trainer' later in this chapter).

Structuring your cardio exercise

You can structure your cardio exercise in two ways: *steady-state exercise* or *interval training*.

- **Steady-state cardiovascular exercise** means that you exercise at a certain pace (or a certain target heart rate), and you stay there for a predetermined length of time. If you're new to exercise, Dan recommends you start with steady-state cardio because it's easier. You don't want to over-stress your joints and muscles with high-intensity exercise that you're not yet conditioned for.

  Your goal should be a cardio workout that lasts somewhere between 10 and 60 minutes, depending on its intensity and your fitness levels. Work at a level of difficulty between 5 (very manageable) and 8 (pretty hard) or use the target heart rate system if you prefer (refer to the preceding section for an explanation of these difficulty levels and target heart rate).

✓ **Interval training** is a more difficult version of cardiovascular exercise. You take a standard steady-state workout and sprinkle in high-intensity intervals of near-maximum effort. With interval training, you get more work done in less time, you burn more kilojoules, you get better fitness benefits and you get a longer *afterburn*, meaning that your metabolism stays elevated for a longer time after your workout.

Here's an example of a 20- to 22-minute cardiovascular workout using interval training:

1. Three minutes at level 3 (very easy) as a warm-up

2. Twenty to sixty seconds of near-maximum work (level 9 to 10)

3. Three minutes at level 5 for recovery

4. Repeat Steps 2 and 3 three more times (four total intervals)

5. Three minutes at level 3 for a cool-down

Dan usually recommends that most people aim to incorporate interval training as soon as they're physically and medically able because it yields more health and fitness benefits, requires shorter workouts, and keeps you from getting bored. However, steady-state workouts are preferable to some people. Maybe you enjoy the peace and meditative state that can come from a steady-state jog or cycling workout. Perhaps you enjoy doing cardio with a friend or a running group and use the time as much for socialising as you do for exercise. Whatever your reason to pick one over the other, the most important things are that you do it, you enjoy it, and you stay consistent with your workouts!

Watching out for trouble

One of the downsides to any repetitive activity (like cardio) is that it leaves you vulnerable to overuse injuries like tendinitis, bursitis and stress fractures. Here are some tips to help you stay injury-free:

✓ **Vary your activity frequently.** Performing a variety of activities utilises the muscles differently and helps limit overuse of any one system. Take a break from the treadmill and use the bike instead. Get outside and play tennis or shoot some basketball. If you're a jogger, mix up your routes so you don't run the same terrain every day. Variety keeps both your body and your brain fresh!

✓ **Recognise signs of overuse.** Stay on the lookout for consistently irritated muscles, reduced physical performance, sluggishness, achy joints or frequent illness. If you experience any of these symptoms, listen to your body and take a few days off to see whether that helps rejuvenate you.

✔ **Stretch regularly throughout the day.** Having certain muscles that are too tight is asking for injury. Get an evaluation from a good physical therapist or qualified exercise professional to find out what you need to stretch and how to do it.

✔ **Don't overdo it.** The key to long-term success is to be consistent, with a gradual progression of overload and physical challenges. Use a sensible progression of increasing time or intensity — don't try to get in shape in a week!

Developing a Strength Training Workout

Strength training — working out with weights or other resistance like your own body weight, exercise tubing, medicine balls, sandbags or suspension straps — increases strength, improves flexibility, raises metabolism, improves immunity, increases bone density, improves balance and day-to-day function, increases insulin response and boosts energy. Plus it's fun!

Choosing the right exercises

A comprehensive strength training program needs to incorporate the six basic types of body movements that utilise all the major muscle groups. Although it's tempting to seek out exercises that target your so-called problem areas, exercising particular muscles doesn't burn fat away from that specific area; that's a myth called *spot reduction*. When your body pulls out fat for fuel, it takes it from wherever it pleases and, unfortunately, you have no control over where that is. Being able to decide where the fat comes off would be great, but your body doesn't work that way. Exercise and proper nutrition make you lose fat, but you can't decide where.

The following list shows the six major types of exercises that should make up the foundation of your strength training workouts. The specific variations and the level of difficulty of these exercises that you choose depend on your abilities and your goals. This is where some professional guidance is beneficial; check out the sidebar 'Finding a fitness trainer' later in the chapter.

✔ **Triple-extension movements** are multi-joint leg exercises like squats, lunges, step-ups and leg presses. They work all the muscles of the thighs and hips.

✔ **Pushing movements** work the chest, shoulders and arms. Examples are push-ups, bench presses and chest flies.

✔ **Pulling movements** work the back, shoulders, neck and arms. Examples are rows, chin-ups, pull-downs and reverse flies. Pulling exercises are essential for correct posture.

✔ **Core exercises** focus on the midsection — waist, trunk and pelvis. A strong core is essential for spinal stability, a strong pelvic floor and the prevention of back injuries. Examples of core exercises are crunches, sit-ups, planks, twists and back extensions.

✔ **Overhead movements**, like the overhead press and the lateral raise, work the shoulders and arms.

✔ **Posterior chain movements** target the group of muscles behind you — the hamstrings, glutes and spinal erectors (the lower back muscles). Exercises that work the posterior chain are dead lifts, bridges and hip extensions.

For more detailed information about what muscles do and which exercises work which muscles, see the *Muscles Overview* article posted on www.dummies.com/extras/beatingsugaraddictionau.

Figuring sets and reps for optimal results

Following are a couple of definitions so that when exercise stuff comes up in conversation with your friends, you can sound like you know what you're talking about.

When you execute an exercise move one time, that's called a *repetition*, or *rep* for short. When you do a bunch of repetitions in a row, that group of reps is called a *set*. Suppose you're doing the Romanian dead lift (see Figure 12-6) for the posterior chain — you do it 12 times before you tire out, you rest a minute, and then you do it another 12 times. The way you describe what you did is to say you did *two sets of 12 reps*. Congratulations — now you sound like a workout veteran!

If you're into fitness magazines or blogs, you'll find a million variations of sets and reps options out there. To simplify things, here are some very basic guidelines for beginners: Start with one set of each of the six basic exercise movements in the preceding section, and pick a weight or a level of difficulty that allows you to perform 15 to 20 repetitions. As your strength and abilities improve, gradually increase both the number of sets and the difficulty of the exercise, and work your way up to three or four sets of 8 to 10 repetitions.

Balancing strength training and recovery time

When you tax your muscles with strength training, they need some time to recover and rebuild. The harder you work your muscles, the more recovery time they need. Give yourself at least 48 hours of recovery between workouts with weights — or more if you're still sore.

Your body makes muscle and bone improvements while you're resting, not while you work out. If you don't give yourself adequate recovery time, you won't get the desired *physiological adaptations*, and you can start to experience signs of overtraining — consistent soreness and fatigue, poor muscular performance and overuse injuries like tendinitis. Being motivated is great, but don't overdo it! For most folks, three 30-minute resistance training workouts each week are plenty.

Performing Basic Strength Training Exercises Correctly

Proper form is important for getting the most out of your strength workouts, and it's also essential for staying free of injuries. In addition to reading through the descriptions and instructions presented in this section, we strongly suggest that you get at least a few lessons from a qualified exercise professional, both to teach you correct execution of the exercises and to determine which variations and levels of difficulty are appropriate for you. See the sidebar 'Finding a fitness trainer' later in this chapter for some tips on seeking out professional exercise instruction.

Exercises for the thighs, glutes and hips

The thighs and hips are some of the largest and strongest muscles in your body. They're responsible for moving you around all day, and they're the driving force when you stand, sit, walk, run, jump, squat down, and go up and down stairs. Keeping your legs strong is especially important for the ageing population to keep good mobility and to prevent falls.

Squat

The *squat* (see Figure 12-1) is one of the fundamental functional exercise moves. More than 200 muscles are active when you do a squat, and it has many practical carry-overs to daily life. You need to master the squat before tackling the more advanced, single-leg moves like lunges or step-ups.

Start with your feet shoulder-width apart and angled out slightly, with your heels planted firmly on the floor. Keeping your back muscles tight and the shape of your spine the same, start to lean your pelvis and upper body forward (keep your chest up) as you begin to bend your knees, like you're starting to sit down into a chair. If you look at yourself from the side, your shoulder should be over your ankle. Continue bending your knees and sinking your hips down until (ideally) your thighs are parallel to the ground. Keep your weight back, press your heels into the floor and drive yourself back up to the standing position.

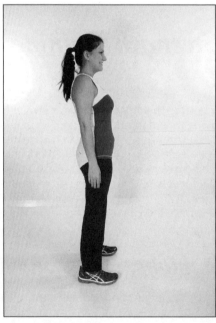 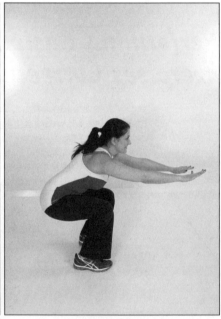

Figure 12-1:
Squat.

Photograph © Shannon Fontaine Photography

 If a full squat (thighs parallel to the floor) is too hard or if you're not flexible enough to get down all the way, stick with a shorter squat — try just half-way down — until your strength and flexibility improve. On the other hand, if squatting with just your body weight gets too easy, hold some dumbbells while you do it or add a five-second hold at the bottom of each rep. Or both!

Feel free to practise this move with some balance assistance until you feel confident; try squatting with your butt against a wall until you feel like you can keep your balance without help. Alternatively, you can try holding onto a chair or a broomstick with your arms while you squat.

Lunge

A *lunge* (see Figure 12-2) is a more difficult version of the squat because most of your weight is on one leg. Begin standing with your feet underneath your hip sockets. Shift your weight onto one leg and slide the other foot approximately 2 feet behind you. Keeping your weight on the heel of your front foot, begin to squat, bending both knees and leaning your upper body forward (just like a squat) so that your shoulder stays over your front ankle. When your back knee touches the floor, press your front heel into the floor and pull yourself forward into the standing position. Be sure to keep your front knee over your ankle — don't let your thigh roll inward. Do some reps on one leg and then switch sides. Don't be surprised if one side is significantly harder than the other.

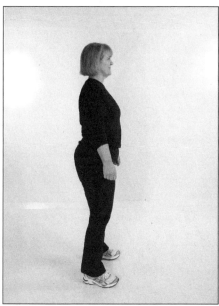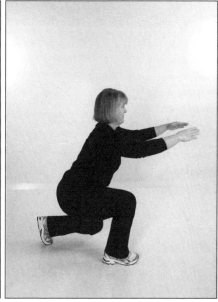

Figure 12-2:
Lunge.

Photograph © Shannon Fontaine Photography

The lunge has many variations, like forward lunges, walking lunges and side lunges. Master this version (stepping back into the lunge position) before you try any others.

Lying hip adduction

The *lying hip adduction* (see Figure 12-3) is an exercise for the inner thigh muscles. Lie on your side, bend your top knee and plant your top foot flat on the floor in front of your bottom knee. Flex your inner thigh muscles on your bottom leg to lift your bottom leg off the ground. Hold for one second and then lower. Repeat reps on one side and then flip over and do the other leg.

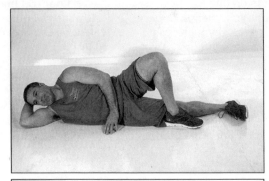

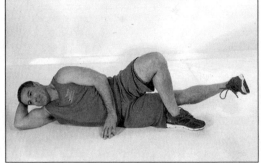

Figure 12-3:
Lying hip
adduction.

Photograph © Shannon Fontaine Photography

Lying hip abduction

The *lying hip abduction* (see Figure 12-4) is the opposite move of the lying hip adduction. Lie on your side with your bottom knee bent and your top leg straight and parallel to your spine (it will feel like it's behind you). Flex your foot (pull your toes up toward your shin) and turn your top thigh one click outward so that your kneecap and foot point a little bit upward instead of straight ahead. Lift your top leg approximately 45 degrees, hold for one second and slowly lower. Do your reps on one hip and then flip over and do the other side. Like the lunge, you'll probably find that one hip is weaker than the other. If that's the case, do one set on the weak side, one set on the stronger side, and a second set on the weaker side to bring it up to snuff.

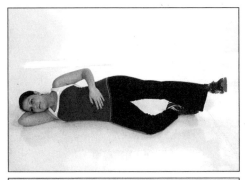

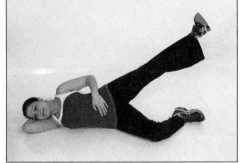

Figure 12-4:
Lying hip
abduction.

Photograph © Shannon Fontaine Photography

Exercises for the posterior chain

Strengthening your hamstrings, glutes and lower back muscles is important for avoiding injury and chronic back pain. Mastering these exercises is also good training for keeping proper spine mechanics when you're lifting things or bending over to pick up stuff.

Bridge

To perform the *bridge* (see Figure 12-5), lie on your back with your knees bent, your heels planted on the floor and your feet flexed up off the ground. Brace your trunk with your core muscles so you can keep your spine from changing shape while you do the move. Press your heels down into the floor to drive your hips up toward the ceiling. Squeeze your glutes (butt muscles) and don't overarch your lower back — the shape of your spine shouldn't change while you bridge. Hold the top of the bridge for one second and then slowly lower.

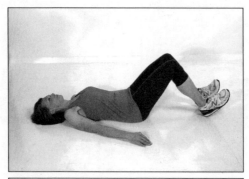

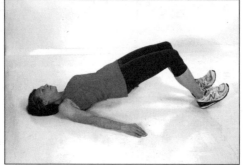

Figure 12-5:
Hamstring
bridge.

Photograph © Shannon Fontaine Photography

More advanced variations of the bridge include putting your feet on an exercise ball or doing the bridge with one leg instead of two. Or, if you're really getting strong, both!

Romanian dead lift

One of Dan's favourite exercises for the posterior chain is the *Romanian dead lift* (see Figure 12-6). It's a very functional, practical exercise for strengthening the back and ingraining proper lifting mechanics.

Holding a pair of dumbbells, start in a standing position with your knees unlocked and your feet about 6 inches apart. Tighten your back muscles to put a little arch in your back, and lean forward from your hips, keeping your back nice and tight. Don't allow your spine to round or your shoulders to hump over. When you can no longer tilt your pelvis any farther (your hamstrings will reach their end range of motion), stop and pull yourself back up to the standing position, using your back muscles.

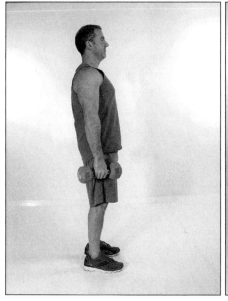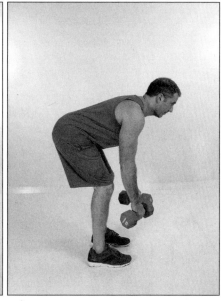

Photograph © Shannon Fontaine Photography

Figure 12-6:
Romanian
dead lift.

Exercises for the shoulders and arms

Keeping your arms and shoulders in good shape helps make you stronger
for your daily activities. Doing so also makes you look great in T-shirts and
sleeveless dresses!

Overhead press

The basic exercise for your shoulders is the *overhead press*
(see Figure 12-7). Start in a standing position with your knees unlocked,
your elbows bent so your forearms are perpendicular to the floor, and
your upper arms at your sides. Drive your arms up to the vertical position
(touchdown!) so your elbows are in line with your ears. Don't overarch
your back; leave your hips over your heels. Slowly lower your elbows back
down to your sides.

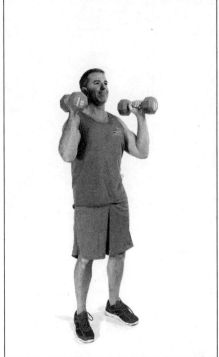 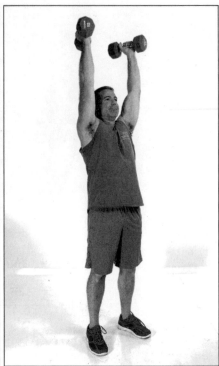

Figure 12-7:
Overhead
press.

Photograph © Shannon Fontaine Photography

Push-ups

Push-ups (see Figure 12-8) are a good way to strengthen your chest, arms and shoulders. Start on your knees with your hands slightly wider than shoulder-width apart. Keep your hips down, creating a straight line between your knees and your head. Bend your elbows and pull your shoulder blades together to lower your body until your chest touches the floor. Your arms should be approximately 45 degrees out from your ribs. Flex your chest and arm muscles to press yourself back to the straight-arm position.

As you get stronger, you can work towards doing push-ups on your toes rather than your knees.

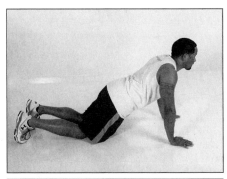

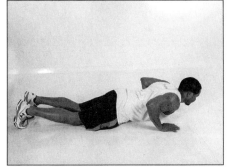

Figure 12-8:
Push-up.

Photograph © Shannon Fontaine Photography

Biceps curl

The *biceps* are the muscles on the front of the upper arm that bend your elbow. To perform the *biceps curl* (see Figure 12-9), start in a standing position holding dumbbells with your palms facing forward. Bend both elbows, pulling your palms toward your shoulders. Try not to let your elbows swing forward at the top; keep them at your ribs. Squeeze your biceps for one second at the top and then slowly straighten your arms right back to the starting position. Straighten your arms all the way at the bottom.

Lying triceps extension

To work the backs of your arms, grab some dumbbells and start the *lying triceps extension* (see Figure 12-10) on your back, with your knees bent and your arms straight up toward the ceiling. Keeping your elbows fixed on an imaginary board or shelf, bend both elbows, lowering your hands to your ears. Be careful not to hit yourself in the head with the weights! Flex your triceps to straighten your arms back to the starting position.

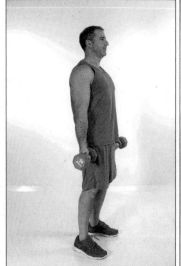
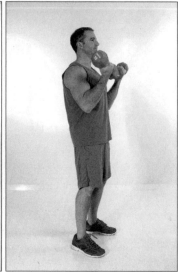

Figure 12-9:
Biceps curl.

Photograph © Shannon Fontaine Photography

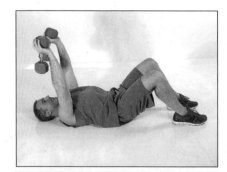
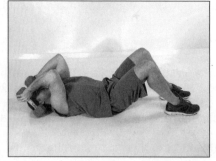

Figure 12-10:
Lying triceps
extension.

Photograph © Shannon Fontaine Photography

Pulling exercises for the back

Keeping the upper back muscles strong is important for good posture and for preventing chronic neck and shoulder pain. Most people who sit a lot need extra work in this area. In your workouts, be sure to do at least as much pulling as you do pushing, if not more.

Standing tubing row

The *standing tubing row* (see Figure 12-11) is a great way to strengthen your upper back and improve your posture. Grab your exercise tubing and insert the anchor into the hinge side of the door. Stand facing the anchor and split your feet so you're braced with one foot ahead of the other. Begin with both arms straight ahead, palms facing each other. Squeeze your shoulder blades together and pull your elbows back, keeping your forearms parallel to the floor. The end position is your shoulder blades squeezed in toward your spine and down away from your ears. Hold the squeeze for one second and then reverse the move back to the starting position.

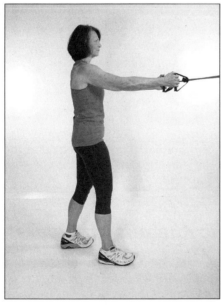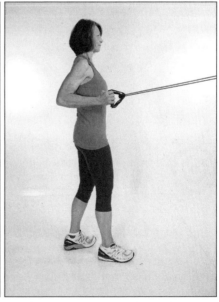

Figure 12-11:
Standing tubing row.

Photograph © Shannon Fontaine Photography

Single-arm row

Another common variation of the row is the *single-arm row* (see Figure 12-12). Start standing with a dumbbell in one hand. Step forward with the opposite leg and lean forward with a straight spine (no rounding), resting the non-dumbbell hand on your forward thigh. Perform the rowing movement on the dumbbell side just like you perform the standing row — pull your shoulder blade back toward your spine and pull your arm back, keeping your forearm perpendicular to the ground. Try not to twist your upper body as you pull. Hold the retracted position for one second and then return to the starting position.

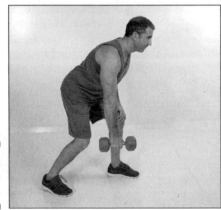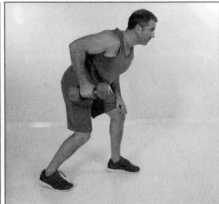

Figure 12-12: Single-arm row.

Photograph © Shannon Fontaine Photography

If you find it too difficult to keep your back correct when doing the leaning-over rowing version, try putting your knee and hand (the nonworking side) on a bench, chair or exercise ball instead.

Core exercises for the abs and waist

Remember that exercising your abdominal muscles doesn't burn fat away from that area! Smart eating and consistent exercise create the physiological environment and caloric deficit needed to lose body fat. You can't pick where your fat comes off, and you can't out-exercise a bad diet!

U crunch

The *U crunch* (see Figure 12-13) is a core exercise that strengthens the abdominals and stretches the lower back. Start by lying on your back with your feet up, your knees bent and your arms up toward the ceiling. Flex your abdominal muscles to curl your spine forward so that your chest and ribs pull down toward your navel and your pelvis rolls back toward your ribs. Aim for half the movement to come from your upper body and half from the pelvis roll. Hold the contracted position for one second and then unroll back to the starting position. Be careful not to overarch your lower back in the starting position.

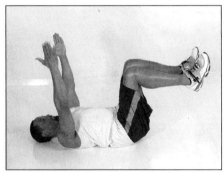

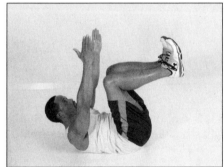

Figure 12-13:
U crunch.

Photograph © Shannon Fontaine Photography

Seated twist

The _seated twist_ (see Figure 12-14) strengthens the waist and targets the twisting muscles — primarily your _obliques_ and _spinal erectors_. Start seated on the floor with your knees bent. Crunch your stomach muscles (pulling your ribs down and rolling your pelvis back) so your lower back is rounded. Rock back onto your tailbone, maintaining a rounded lower back. Slowly twist your upper body approximately 45 degrees from side to side until you can't hold the position anymore. If your back hurts before your abs, you've lost your rounded shape. If just body weight is too easy, hold a medicine ball or dumbbell while you twist.

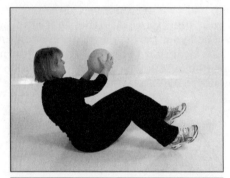

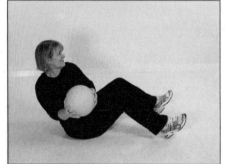

Figure 12-14:
Seated
twist.

Photograph © Shannon Fontaine Photography

Plank

The *plank* (see Figure 12-15) is one of the mainstays of core stabilisation exercises. The goal is to be able to stiffen your spine like a board or a plank and hold it in the same shape in a variety of positions.

To begin the basic plank, start on all fours (hands and knees) and then walk your hands forward until the line between your knees and your head is straight (like a plank). Flex your abdominal muscles and roll your pelvis under so your lower back is rounded. Hold your spine in that shape and go down onto your elbows where your hands were. Just hold still and breathe. Feel your abs?

If you can hold this position for 15 seconds and it's not difficult, lift up onto your toes instead of your knees (see Figure 12-15). Just like in the seated twist, if your back hurts instead of your abs, you've lost your rounded lower back. Work up to being able to stay in the plank position for 60 seconds.

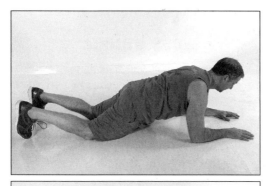

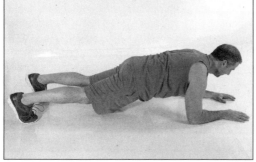

Figure 12-15:
Plank on
knees and
toes.

Photograph © Shannon Fontaine Photography

 A common variation of this exercise is the *side plank* (see Figure 12-16). Start lying on your side with your feet stacked on top of each other and your bottom forearm on the floor. Lift your hips to form a straight line from feet to head.

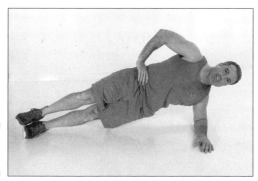

Figure 12-16:
Side plank.

Photograph © Shannon Fontaine Photography

Finding a fitness trainer

Because everyone's body is different and everyone learns differently, we recommend that you hire a qualified exercise instructor to help you put together a safe and effective exercise program to reach your goals.

You can find multitudes of gyms and private exercise studios, all of which have fitness trainers available. Sadly, the fact that someone holds a fitness certification doesn't mean that he or she is a well-educated, qualified teacher. Instead of hiring just anyone, do some homework first to make sure that you find the best teacher available in your area.

If you know some local health and wellness providers (massage therapists, physicians, chiropractors or physical therapists), ask whom they'd recommend for fitness instruction. Barring that, call some personal trainers and ask, 'If I can't work with you (or someone in your company), whom do you suggest I hire?' If you get the same name more than once, chances are you have a winner.

To make a blanket statement, if you need help with basic fitness programming (losing weight and getting in shape), your trainer should put you on a system relatively similar to what we've outlined in this chapter. If you're new to exercise and your personal trainer starts you off with a bodybuilding-style split routine on your first week (chest and arms on one day, legs on another day, and so on), find a different trainer who's more versed in functional fitness and modern exercise programming.

Putting It All Together: Sample Workouts

You can do countless variations of workouts, so you'll never be bored! This section includes two examples to get you started: An easy workout and a difficult one.

Example workout 1 (easy)

Warm-up: Five to ten minutes of light activity of your choice — for example, treadmill, elliptical, seated rowing machine, stationary bike or marching in place.

Strength training portion: One set of 15 to 20 repetitions of each of these six exercises, with approximately one minute rest in between sets:

1. Squats

2. Push-ups

3. Standing rows with tubing

4. Bridges

5. Overhead presses with dumbbells

6. Planks or U crunches

Cardiovascular portion: 20 to 30 minutes of the cardio exercise of your choice at low to medium intensity: 60 to 75 per cent of (208 – 70 per cent of your age).

Five-minute cool-down: Low-intensity version of the cardio you were doing, or just walking.

Flexibility: Stretch your three or four tightest areas for 30 seconds, two times each. Don't forget to breathe!

Example workout 2 (difficult)

Warm-up: Five to ten minutes of light activity of your choice — for example, treadmill, elliptical, seated rowing machine, stationary bike or marching in place.

Strength training portion: Perform one set of 8 to 10 repetitions of each of these six exercises, with very little rest between exercises. When you've gone through all six, rest for about two minutes and then repeat the list. After two rounds, see whether you have a third round in you!

1. Lunges (8 to 10 on each leg)

2. Push-ups

3. Single-arm rows with dumbbell (8 to 10 each side)

4. Romanian dead lifts

5. Dumbbell curls into overhead presses

6. Seated twists with a medicine ball or dumbbell

Cardiovascular portion: Fifteen minutes of the cardio exercise of your choice at medium to high intensity: 75 to 90 per cent of (208 – 70 per cent of your age).

Five-minute cool-down: Low-intensity version of the cardio you were doing, or just walking.

Flexibility: Stretch your three or four tightest areas for 30 seconds, two times each. Don't forget to breathe!

Optimal wellness includes both good nutrition and exercise. You can't exercise off a bad diet!

Part IV
Sugar-Busting Recipes

Five Easy Substitutions for Healthier Eating

- **Drink mineral water instead of soft drinks.** Mineral water flavoured with citrus will give you the fizz and the flavour that you love without the sugar and chemicals that come with soft drinks. Staying hydrated can help stave off sugar cravings too!

- **Eat a protein-based snack for morning tea and afternoon tea.** Seeds and nuts, cottage or ricotta cheese and Greek plain yoghurt are all blood-stabilising, yet filling snacks. Eating a small protein-rich snack will keep the sugar monster quiet.

- **Snack on raw veggies instead of junk food.** Keeping fresh raw veggies ready to snack on will make it easy for you to make the smart choice when you need to nibble. Crunching on low-calorie, high-nutrient vegetables will satisfy your hunger, and add valuable fibre, antioxidants and nutrition to your daily diet.

- **Choose whole grains like oats, rice and spelt instead of white flour.** Whole grains are loaded with B-vitamins and minerals. The fibre from whole grains helps you feel full and helps keep your blood sugar and insulin levels from spiking too fast. White flour digests quickly and causes a more rapid rise in blood sugar, followed by a sugar crash that leads to hunger and cravings.

- **Buy pasture-raised eggs and meat instead of feedlot products.** Animals raised in commercial feedlots are kept in overcrowded conditions and are fed industrial feed containing chemicals and antibiotics. Quality food is your greatest wellness insurance — if you can afford it, buy it.

Check out www.dummies.com/extras/beatingsugaraddictionau for more sugar-busting tips and tricks.

In this part . . .

- ✔ Start the day off right by going beyond the cereal box with protein-packed, low-sugar breakfasts.

- ✔ Prevent midday slumps by making smart lunch choices loaded with veggies and healthy protein.

- ✔ Fortify your family with speedy dinner recipes ranging from creative seafood options to more traditional meat and vegetarian dishes.

- ✔ Satisfy cravings with healthy snacks that fill you up without sabotaging your low-sugar goals.

- ✔ Redefine desserts to get the satisfaction you want with less sugar and more flavour.

Chapter 13

Energy-Boosting Breakfasts

An old saying advises, 'Eat breakfast like a king, lunch like a prince, and dinner like a pauper', but many Australians and New Zealanders do the opposite. Undereating during the day and overeating at night is exactly the wrong way to eat if you're trying to lose weight. Doing so also works against you if you're trying to keep your energy up and your mental performance sharp. When you wake up in the morning, you've gone eight or ten hours without food, your body is craving nourishment, and your brain needs glucose to function at its best. Skipping breakfast is one of the worst possible things you can do — you set yourself up for fatigue, poor mental acuity and sugar cravings later in the day.

In this chapter, we take you through the benefits of a good breakfast, and provide some tasty low-sugar options.

Appreciating the Importance of Breakfast

People who eat breakfast are far more likely to get a healthy intake of vitamins and minerals than those who don't. In one recent study, researchers found that people who ate a hearty breakfast containing more than 25 per cent of their daily calories had a higher intake of essential vitamins and minerals — and lower cholesterol levels too!

Thinking outside the cereal box

Be wary of packaged cereals! When some people sit down for breakfast, they automatically grab a quick, all-carbohydrate food like breakfast cereal or a muffin. Don't be afraid to think outside the sugary breakfast food box. A much healthier choice would be eggs and bacon, but you have so many more options to consider. A traditional Japanese breakfast consists of a small piece of fish (like salmon), some light vegetables, and a tiny portion of rice accompanied by a small bowl of miso soup. The health benefits of fish and vegetables in the morning are huge, and the omega-3 fats (refer to Chapter 5) in salmon are terrific for your skin, help regulate mood, and are essential for proper hormone formation. If breakfasting on fish or other leftovers is too much of a stretch for you, consider these options:

- **A cup of organic Greek yoghurt with nuts, grapes or berries:** Greek yoghurt contains active probiotic cultures (beneficial bacteria — refer to Chapter 5) and has twice the protein and half the carbs as regular yoghurt. Also consider A2 milk and plain yoghurt for their nutritional properties.

- **Natural peanut or almond butter on a slice of wholegrain bread:** Fold it in half and enjoy your easy, no-cook breakfast. A nut butter sandwich goes great with a cup of English breakfast or green tea.

- **Smoked salmon with avocado on a slice of rye bread:** This gives you quality protein, fat and long-lasting carbs without any sugar.

- **Goat's cheese and avocado on toasted spelt bread:** This is another way to get lots of good energy and nutrients without added sugar.

- **A 'clean' whey protein shake:** It's fast, inexpensive and versatile, and has the protein you may be used to getting from bacon, sausage and eggs. Try frozen berries or half a cup of frozen banana with powdered whey and a quarter cup of coconut, almond, organic, A2 or rice milk, and some water. Adding a teaspoon of flax oil, chia seeds, coconut butter or some avocado to the shake adds essential fats and helps the smoothie 'stick' with you a little longer. Experiment and see what you like!

If you still feel you'd like a cereal option, make sure you choose one with a low-sugar content. Always read the nutritional panel and ingredients label. Check out www.howmuchsugar. com for David Gillespie's list of best cereal choices by sugar content (available to members only — you have to pay a small annual fee to access most of the lists and guides on David's site, but this gives you access to some great information).

Research shows that one out of four Australians and New Zealanders skip breakfast, and many kids leave for school without it. The implications are dramatic, both physically and mentally. People who skip breakfast are more than four times as likely to be obese than people who eat something in the morning. Skipping breakfast makes you fatter and foggier!

Numerous studies over the years have shown that skipping breakfast affects the behaviour and mental performance of children in school too. Kids who eat breakfast have better memory, and higher maths and reading scores. Kids who are hungry or have blood sugar swings have a higher number of behaviour problems, including difficulty with friends and teachers, acknowledging rules, concentrating and moody behaviour. This all leads to feeling poorly about themselves. A sad and vicious cycle we see often with children, and families who believe their child has ADHD, is often simply caused by poor eating.

Launching Your Day the Low-Sugar Way

The traditional breakfast for most Aussies and Kiwis is typically an all-carbohydrate affair. Breakfast is often loaded with muffins, cakes, breakfast cereals and pastries that cause a giant rush of sugar into the body, with the corresponding insulin crash several hours later. Do you ever feel sleepy after a meal like this? If you do, imagine how your kids might feel.

The ideal breakfast has a high-protein content. Higher-protein breakfasts translate into a more sustained level of energy throughout the morning (no carb crash). Protein fills you up longer, meaning you're less likely to have midmorning cravings. You're also less likely to overeat at lunch or to get so hungry during the day that you grab whatever is available in the break room or the vending machine. More protein at breakfast also increases metabolism; in one study, a high-protein breakfast *doubled* the metabolism of healthy young women!

Traditional protein sources for breakfast include eggs, bacon or ham (choose nitrate-free, if possible), sausage, cheese, yoghurt, smoked salmon, tofu, raw seeds and nuts, and whey. You have plenty of other options, though — don't get stuck in a breakfast rut!

We believe that food should always come before a supplementary protein powder but if you need additional protein, are recovering from an illness, or need something quick yet satisfying, a good quality protein powder is fine. The subject of what makes a good quality protein powder can be quite controversial and the debate around the best powder to choose is in depth. Keep things simple by choosing a 'clean' whey protein powder, which can be a beneficial addition to your healthy food choices. (Refer to Chapter 5 for guidelines on what constitutes a 'clean' protein powder.)

Don't eat the same thing for breakfast every day. Eating a variety of foods means that you get a wider spectrum of nutrients. Changing up the breakfast routine also makes the meal more appealing — especially if you don't like to eat in the morning.

Eggs: Good or bad?

Some published research has concluded that the consumption of eggs (or red meat) raises your risk of cardiovascular disease — atherosclerosis, heart attacks, strokes and so on. After reviewing the current research available and having an understanding of how the body's inflammatory response affects the cardiovascular system, we believe the questioning of these foods is based on the quality and origin of the food itself.

Eating food produced from sick animals that are fed chemically enhanced, genetically modified grain raises the level of inflammation in your body. Garbage in, garbage out as they say. The profile for healthy animal products (organic and pasture-fed) is more nutritious, and these foods don't cause the high inflammatory response that the industrial feedlot products do.

Crowded living conditions are the reason commercial producers use antibiotics in their chicken feed and why industrial eggs must be bathed in chemicals to sanitise them. We recommend pasture-fed, antibiotic-free eggs because pasture feeding gives eggs a higher nutrient content than conventional eggs, is better for the chickens, and doesn't perpetuate antibiotic resistance like conventional chicken feed does.

Eggs are loaded with protein and other nutrients, such as phosphatidylcholine for the brain and lutein and zeaxanthin for the eyes, and guess what? Eggs have no sugar. If you need to lower the amount of fat in your diet, you can use egg whites instead of whole eggs, but if you do, remember that you're missing out on a lot of important nutrients in the pasture-fed yolks.

Grab 'n' Go Coconut Muffins

Prep time: 10 min • **Cook time:** 20–25 min • **Yield:** 6 muffins

Ingredients	Directions
6 eggs	*1* Preheat the oven to 180 degrees Celsius. In a muffin pan, line 6 cups with paper muffin liners.
¼ cup coconut butter, melted	
½ cup extra-virgin olive oil	*2* In a large mixing bowl, beat together the eggs, coconut butter and olive oil with an electric mixer on low speed.
½ cup coconut flour	
1 tablespoon rosemary, thyme or sage (for a savoury muffin)	*3* Add the flour, herbs, baking powder and sea salt. Beat well on medium speed.
¼ teaspoon baking powder	
½ teaspoon sea salt	*4* Spoon the batter into the prepared muffin pan. Bake for 20 to 25 minutes, or until brown and firm to the touch.
	5 Cool on wire racks.

Per serving: *Kilojoules 1465/Calories 350 (From Fat 283); Fat 31.5g (Saturated 12.6g); Cholesterol 186mg; Sodium 285mg; Carbohydrate 7.4g (Dietary Fibre 4.2g); Protein 7.6g; Sugar 3.9g.*

Tip: To make sweet muffins, replace herbs with 1 teaspoon of cinnamon or chia spices (see www.hariharchai.com.au or www.thespicetradingcompany.com.au for amazing spices), and/or ½ teaspoon of pure vanilla.

Source: *Adapted from recipe by www.ahealthyview.com.*

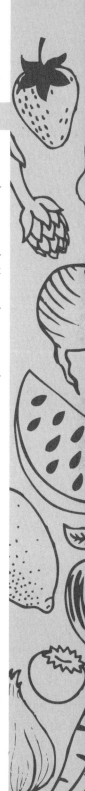

Almond and Buckwheat Pancakes

Prep time: 5 min • **Cook time:** 10 min • **Yield:** 4 servings (6–8 large pancakes, or 24 pikelets)

Ingredients	Directions
1 cup organic buckwheat flour (or ½ cup buckwheat and ½ cup wholemeal spelt flour)	*1* Whisk the buckwheat flour, spelt flour (if using), chia seeds, almond meal and baking powder together in a large mixing bowl with a balloon whisk.
1 tablespoon chia seeds	
2 tablespoons almond meal or flour	*2* Add the egg and most of the milk and whisk until combined. If mixture seems thick, whisk through the rest of the milk. Don't over-mix or you will toughen the batter.
1 teaspoon baking powder	
1 egg	*3* Lightly butter and heat a heavy fry pan to medium heat.
1 cup milk	
Butter for cooking	*4* Spoon the batter onto the hot fry pan in 7- to 10-centimetre diameter pancakes, and cook until bubbles form (2 to 3 minutes). Flip the pancakes with a spatula and continue cooking until golden brown on both sides, about 2 minutes more.
Dash of cinnamon	
	5 Turn on to a plate with a paper towel. Stack them up and, if not eating immediately, keep warm in an oven (cover with foil to keep moist and soft).
	6 Serve with butter and a sprinkle of cinnamon.

Per serving: Kilojoules 900/Calories 215 (From Fat 70); Fat 7.9g (Saturated 3.4g); Cholesterol 58mg; Sodium 180mg; Carbohydrate 27.5g (Dietary Fibre 4.9g); Protein 5.8g; Sugar 0.9g.

Tip: Depending on what flour you use, you may need to increase the milk a bit. Also, chia seeds swell on sitting, which again may mean you need to add more milk.

Vary It! Substitute some of the milk with sour cream or buttermilk to make the pancakes lighter and fluffier.

Vary It! Add ingredients such as a tablespoon of vanilla essence or walnut oil, or a tablespoon of wheat germ to change the flavour of the pancakes or boost the fibre and nutrient content.

Source: Adapted from recipe by Cindy Luken www.lukbeautifood.com.

Muesli

Prep time: 12 min • **Yield:** 12 servings (1 cup each)

Ingredients	Directions
4½ cups traditional rolled oats (not instant)	**1** Combine all ingredients except the almond milk in a large mixing bowl. Mix well and transfer to an airtight container for storage.
½ cup toasted wheat germ	
½ cup oat bran	**2** To prepare the muesli hot, add the almond milk and microwave in a glass container for 90 seconds, stirring once; stir well, add a bit more milk (if required) and enjoy. To prepare the muesli cold, just add the milk and mix it up with a spoon.
2 scoops unsweetened whey protein powder (optional)	
2 tablespoons chia seeds (optional)	
¼ cup sultanas	
¼ cup dried cranberries	
½ cup chopped walnuts	
⅓ cup almond milk, per serving	

Per serving: Kilojoules 1306/Calories 312 (From Fat 69); Fat 7.8g (Saturated 1.2g); Cholesterol 0mg; Sodium 2mg; Carbohydrate 49.8g (Dietary Fibre 8.7g); Protein 12.8g; Sugar 3.6g.

Vary It! Instead of walnuts, substitute ¼ cup sunflower seeds or pumpkin seeds for extra calcium and zinc.

Tip: You can also use unsweetened almond (or other types of) milk.

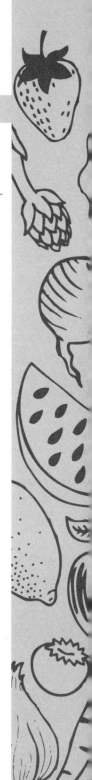

Egg Casserole

Prep time: 20 min, plus refrigeration time • **Cook time:** 50–65 min • **Yield:** 8 servings

Ingredients	Directions
Butter to grease baking dish	*1* Butter a large baking dish.
500 grams ground sausage (available from your local butcher) or chopped chipolatas	*2* Brown the sausage in a fry pan over medium heat, draining fat as needed.
5 slices of wholegrain bread, torn into pieces	*3* Spread the torn bread, cheese and cooked sausage evenly in a pan.
1½ cups grated tasty cheese	
9 large eggs	*4* In a large bowl, beat the eggs well. Add the mustard and then the milk.
1½ teaspoons dry mustard	
3 cups milk	*5* Pour the mixture over the dry ingredients in the pan and refrigerate overnight.
	6 Preheat the oven to 180 degrees Celsius. Bake 45 to 60 minutes, or until the entire casserole is puffed all over.
	7 After removing from the oven, allow the casserole to rest for 5 minutes before serving.

Per serving: Kilojoules 2022/Calories 483 (From Fat 180); Fat 20g (Saturated 13g); Cholesterol 233mg; Sodium 594mg; Carbohydrate 19g (Dietary Fibre 4g); Protein 23g; Sugar 5.9g.

Tip: Buy eggs from pasture-fed chickens from a local farmer who can guarantee that you're getting chemical-free eggs.

Vary It! Serve with a side of spinach or avocado for a well-rounded breakfast.

Breakfast Bowl

Prep time: 20 min • **Cook time:** 15 min • **Yield:** 4 servings

Ingredients	Directions
3 egg whites **1 egg yolk**	**1** Whisk egg whites and yolk together until combined, light and fluffy.
1 teaspoon coconut oil **80 grams sliced smoked salmon**	**2** Heat a small omelette pan and add the oil. Pour in egg mixture and stir with wooden spoon until eggs are lightly scrambled.
½ cup smashed avocado **4 tablespoons tomato salsa (see following recipe)**	**3** Place scrambled eggs on serving plate or bowl, top with smashed avocado and salsa, and place a rosette of smoked salmon on top.

Tomato Salsa

2 egg tomatoes, quartered, seeded and finely chopped **1 green onion, thinly sliced** **2 teaspoons lime juice** **2 teaspoons finely chopped coriander**	**1** Combine all ingredients in a bowl then season to taste with salt and pepper.

Per serving: Kilojoules 620/Calories 148 (From Fat 90); Fat 10g (Saturated 2.7g); Cholesterol 50mg; Sodium 448mg; Carbohydrate 6.8g (Dietary Fibre 4.2g); Protein 8.5g; Sugar 1.5g.

Source: Adapted from recipe by Thr1ve.me.

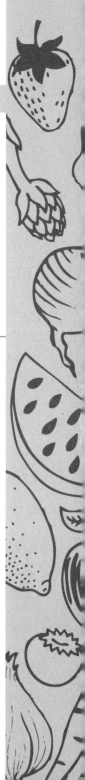

Breakfast Quinoa

Prep time: 10 min • **Cook time:** 20 min • **Yield:** 4 servings

Ingredients	*Directions*
2 cups milk (regular or almond) 1 cup organic quinoa	*1* Pour the milk into a medium saucepan. Add the quinoa, salt and cinnamon and bring to a boil, stirring occasionally.
½ teaspoon salt 1 teaspoon ground cinnamon	*2* Reduce the heat to low, cover and simmer for 15 minutes.
1 teaspoon vanilla extract 5 pitted figs or dates, chopped	*3* When the quinoa is plumped, remove it from the heat.
¼ cup chopped roasted almonds	*4* Stir in the vanilla, figs and almonds. Serve warm.

Per serving: Kilojoules 1164/Calories 278 (From Fat 60); Fat 6.8g (Saturated 0.7g); Cholesterol 2mg; Sodium 344mg; Carbohydrate 42.5g (Dietary Fibre 5g); Protein 12g; Sugar 12.4g.

Tip: To reduce the sugar content, use minimal amount of figs or dates.

Vary It! For added flavour, add a drizzle of local honey or 1 tablespoon of organic butter to Step 4.

Vary It! Add a teaspoon of coconut butter and ½ teaspoon of cinnamon to Step 4.

Egg Tacos

Prep time: 15 min • **Cook time:** 5 min • **Yield:** 8 servings

Ingredients	Directions
4 large eggs **Splash of milk**	*1* In a medium bowl, crack the eggs and add a splash of milk. Beat well and then add the chopped onions.
¼ cup diced red onion **8 corn taco shells (baked not fried)**	*2* Heat the taco shells in a toaster oven until slightly warm.
1 tablespoon butter **4 tablespoons sour cream**	*3* In a medium fry pan, melt the butter over medium heat and then add the egg mixture.
½ cup grated tasty cheese (or cheese of your choice) **1 tomato, chopped**	*4* Scramble the eggs in the skillet, mixing almost constantly. Cook for 3 to 4 minutes, until the eggs are thickened but still moist. Don't overcook.
1 avocado, chopped (optional)	*5* Remove the eggs from the heat immediately and place them in a clean bowl.
	6 Coat the inside of each taco shell with sour cream to taste. Spoon approximately 2 tablespoons of egg and 1 tablespoon of cheese into each shell. Add the tomato and avocado (if desired) to taste.

Per serving: Kilojoules 674/Calories 161 (From Fat 95); Fat 11g (Saturated 4g); Cholesterol 113mg; Sodium 258mg; Carbohydrate 11g (Dietary Fibre 1.5g); Protein 7g; Sugar 1.5g.

Vary It! For a little extra zing, add a dash of hot sauce to your taco or substitute diced jalapeños for the red onions.

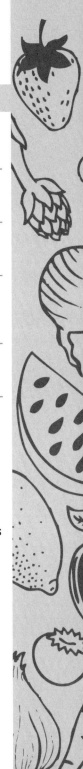

Vegetable Frittata

Prep time: 15 min • **Cook time:** 30–40 min • **Yield:** 8 servings

Ingredients	Directions
2 teaspoons melted butter **24 large eggs** **¼ cup milk** **Juice of 1 lemon** **Olive oil** **1 cup diced capsicum (mix red, green and yellow)** **2 cups chopped fresh spinach** **½ cup diced red onion** **1 cup diced mushrooms (any variety)** **Salt and ground black pepper** **1 cup grated or diced cheese of your choice (feta, goat or tasty)**	*1* Preheat the oven to 180 degrees Celsius. Coat a large cake pan or glass baking dish with butter. Make sure it's well-coated or the frittata will be difficult to get out of the pan.
	2 In a large bowl, whisk together 8 whole eggs, 16 egg whites, milk and lemon juice.
	3 Coat a large fry pan with olive oil and heat over medium-high heat. Sauté the mixed capsicum and onion for 3 to 4 minutes, stirring often. Add the mushrooms and mix thoroughly. Add salt and pepper to taste, and sauté until the capsicum is just tender, about 2 more minutes. Add the spinach and cook until just wilted. Remove from the heat and drain off any remaining water or oil.
	4 Add the vegetables and cheese to the egg mix and stir. Pour the mixture into the cake pan or baking dish. Sprinkle with salt and pepper.
	5 Bake for 20 to 30 minutes, until the eggs are cooked and the cheese is melted. This dish is delicious hot or cold.

Per serving: Kilojoules 1285/Calories 306 (From Fat 176); Fat 19.6g (Saturated 8.5g); Cholesterol 577mg; Sodium 434mg; Carbohydrate 5.6g (Dietary Fibre 0.8g); Protein 22.6g; Sugar 3.6g.

Vary It! Add herbs such as flat-leaf parsley or coriander to Step 4 for added flavour and antioxidants.

High-Protein Oatmeal

Prep time: 5 min • **Cook time:** 10 min • **Yield:** 4 servings

Ingredients	Directions
Pinch of sea salt 2 cups water	*1* In a medium saucepan, add the salt to the water and bring to a boil over high heat.
1 cup traditional oats 2 scoops unsweetened whey protein powder (40 grams) (optional)	*2* Add the oats and reduce the heat to medium. Cook for approximately 5 minutes (until all the water is absorbed), stirring frequently.
¼ cup milk (regular or almond) ½ teaspoon ground cinnamon	*3* Cover and remove from heat. Let stand for 1 to 2 minutes.
½ cup chopped walnuts ½ ripe banana	*4* In a large bowl, combine the cooked oats, whey powder, milk, cinnamon and walnuts. Mix thoroughly.
	5 Serve in two large bowls, topped with banana slices. (If the milk cools down the oatmeal, microwave each bowl for 30 seconds before serving.)

Per serving: Kilojoules 2223/Calories 531 (From Fat 206); Fat 23g (Saturated 2.8g); Cholesterol <1mg; Sodium 314mg; Carbohydrate 64.5g (Dietary Fibre 11.3g); Protein 19g; Sugar 5.9g.

Vary It! Substitute the banana for a handful of berries for a lower sugar option.

Vary It! Add a teaspoon each of sesame, pumpkin and sunflower seeds for additional calcium, zinc and fibre.

Vary It! Add a teaspoon of coconut butter for taste and long-lasting satiation.

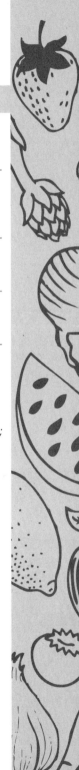

Two-Minute High-Protein Breakfast Smoothie

Ingredients	Directions
1 heaped scoop of clean protein powder **200 millilitres water** **2–3 ice cubes** **¼ ripe avocado** **3 strawberries (or ¼ cup mixed berries)** **½ banana**	*1* Just throw all ingredients in the blender, blend for 30 seconds and enjoy.

Per serving: Kilojoules 1168/Calories 279 (From Fat 155); Fat 8.2g (Saturated 1.6g); Cholesterol 30mg; Sodium 133mg; Carbohydrate 18.3g (Dietary Fibre 4g); Protein 26.1g; Sugar 13.2.

Source: Adapted from recipe by www.180nutrition.com.au.

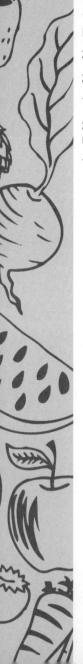

Chapter 14

Powerful Lunches

In This Chapter

▶ Taking your lunch to work

▶ Making some tasty and nutritious lunch recipes

Lunch is the make-or-break meal that determines what you'll feel like during the rest of the day. Poor choices at lunch leave you with low energy for the afternoon and an unstoppable appetite by the time dinner rolls around.

Undereating during the day is one of the primary triggers for sugar cravings at night. Be sure that your daytime meals contain lots of protein and fibre to help keep you satiated and energised for the afternoon.

A low-sugar lunch doesn't have to be a dreary sandwich or salad! Instead, use lunch as an opportunity to experience new and exciting foods. In this chapter, we provide some unconventional low-sugar lunch recipes featuring lamb, tuna, quinoa, edamame and loads of fresh, colourful vegetables. Using these examples, you can experiment with some new flavours and textures and make lunchtime a culinary adventure to spice up your day.

Thirst is one of the things that can trigger a sugar craving. Use lunchtime as a reminder to evaluate how much water you've had so far in the day. By halfway through the day, you should have consumed at least one litre of water.

Some people who are trying to come off sugar and reduce their weight feel hungry, tired or both by around 4 pm. This is the danger time — when everything you have done well can come undone. Almost always, these feelings are due to an inadequate lunch. So if you find yourself hungry or lagging in the afternoon, check what you've eaten. Did you include quality proteins, some good fats, and a small amount of complex carbohydrates (logs; for more on this, refer to Chapter 1) for a proper lunch meal? If not, it could be your biggest downfall.

BYO Lunch

The healthiest people we know have some nutritional traits in common and one of them is 'cook once, eat twice'. Don't forget to make enough in your evening meal so you can have dinner for lunch the next day. It makes your life and nutritional decisions easy. Always go for ease!

If you're not at home during the day, bringing your lunch (and sugar-free snacks) means you're supplied with healthy food throughout the day. Here are some tips for planning and packing your lunch:

- ✔ **Plan ahead.** When cooking fish, chicken or meat for dinner, make some extra for a sandwich or salad for lunch the next day. Roast vegetables can easily be tossed into a salad.

- ✔ **Buy a small esky or chilly bin.** If you don't have access to a refrigerator at work (or if you spend your day in the car), stock an esky or chilly bin with healthy food each morning.

- ✔ **Purchase a wide-mouth thermos.** After you warm this little treasure up in the morning, pop in your leftover soup, casserole or stir-fry from last night's dinner to enjoy for lunch.

- ✔ **If you'll need to heat your food, pack it in glass containers, not plastic.** When plastics get heated, chemicals like *diethylhexyl adipate*, *phthalates* and *Bisphenol A* (BPA) leach out of the plastic. Although the chemicals released from plastics labelled as 'microwave safe' are reported to be a tiny, 'safe' amount, these chemicals are proven carcinogens and endocrine disruptors. We suggest you don't expose yourself or your family to them if you don't have to.

- ✔ **Seek out a healthy takeaway.** Spend some time finding a place close to work that has healthy alternatives for lunch. The world is moving in this direction and plenty of options are now available; you just need to investigate and ask around.

Tuna-Stuffed Tomatoes

Prep time: 10 min • **Cook time:** 8–10 min • **Yield:** 2 servings

Ingredients	Directions
185-gram can tuna in water	**1** Preheat the oven or toaster oven to 175 degrees Celsius.
2 tablespoons chopped cucumber	
2 tablespoons chopped red onion	**2** Drain the tuna and combine it with the cucumber, onion, celery, olive oil, mayonnaise, lemon juice and herbs in a medium bowl. Salt and pepper to taste, and stir together thoroughly with a spoon.
2 tablespoons chopped celery	
1 tablespoon olive oil	
2 tablespoons whole egg mayonnaise	**3** Cut the tomatoes in half horizontally. With a paring knife and spoon, core the tomatoes by scooping out approximately 75 per cent of the insides. Discard the tomato innards.
1 teaspoon fresh-squeezed lemon juice	
1 teaspoon chopped fresh parsley	**4** Fill the cored tomatoes with tuna salad and place them on a baking sheet. Heat them in the oven for 8 to 10 minutes, until the tomatoes are tender and the tuna is warm.
1 teaspoon chopped fresh dill (optional)	
Salt and ground black pepper to taste	
2 large tomatoes	

Per serving: Kilojoules 1113/Calories 266 (From Fat 109); Fat 12.2g (Saturated 1.9g); Cholesterol 31mg; Sodium 432mg; Carbohydrate 13.3g (Dietary Fibre 2.6g); Protein 25.6g; Sugar 7.4g.

Vary It! Add a sprinkling of grated Parmesan cheese to each stuffed tomato before heating.

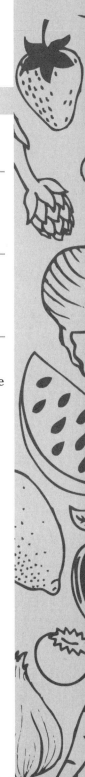

Quinoa and Edamame Salad

Prep time: 10 min • **Cook time:** 25 min • **Yield:** 3–4 servings

Ingredients	Directions
1 cup quinoa **2 cups vegetable broth** **2 cups (about 300 grams) frozen shelled edamame, thawed** **1 cup chopped fresh mushrooms** **1 lemon** **2 tablespoons chopped fresh tarragon (or 2 teaspoons dried)** **2 tablespoons olive oil** **Salt and ground black pepper to taste** **¼ cup chopped walnuts** **2 cups fresh spinach or romaine lettuce**	**1** Rinse the quinoa in a sieve or fine strainer. Toast the quinoa in a dry fry pan over medium heat for 5 to 10 minutes, stirring often. Remove from heat when the quinoa begins to crackle. **2** After the quinoa toasts for approximately 5 minutes, pour the vegetable broth into a large saucepan or small stockpot and bring it to a boil over high heat. **3** Add the quinoa to the boiling broth and return it to a boil. Cover, reduce heat and simmer for about 8 minutes (the quinoa won't be fully cooked). **4** Add the edamame and mushrooms. Cover and cook for 8 minutes longer, until the edamame and quinoa are tender. **5** Halve the lemon and squeeze juice from one half (about 2 tablespoons) into a small bowl. Add the tarragon, olive oil, salt and pepper, and whisk together. **6** Pour the lemon seasoning mix into the quinoa pot and add the walnuts. Mix thoroughly with a fork. **7** Plate each salad with a bed of spinach or lettuce. Scoop the edamame/quinoa mix onto each bed. Squeeze the remaining lemon juice over the top.

Per serving: Kilojoules 1632/Calories 390 (From Fat 12); Fat 3.5g (Saturated 0.5g); Cholesterol 0mg; Sodium 44mg; Carbohydrate 12g (Dietary Fibre 2.5g); Protein 5g; Sugar 3.3g.

Note: This salad is delicious warm or cold.

Vary It! If you're not a fan of edamame, substitute peas or legumes at the end of cooking.

Chicken Broccoli Salad

Prep time: 10 min plus refrigeration time • **Cook time:** 10 min • **Yield:** 4 servings

Ingredients	*Directions*
2 teaspoons cold pressed or extra-virgin olive oil	*1* Coat a small fry pan with olive oil and heat it over medium-high heat.
1 boneless, skinless chicken breast (about 150 grams)	
¼ cup apple cider vinegar	*2* Chop the chicken breast into bite-sized pieces and sauté until browned, about 10 minutes. Stir often.
¾ cup whole egg mayonnaise	
3 cups chopped broccoli	*3* In a small bowl, whisk the vinegar and mayonnaise together until well blended.
½ cup chopped walnuts, almonds or pine nuts	
1 cup shredded carrots	*4* In a large bowl, mix the broccoli, walnuts, carrots, apple and cranberries.
½ Fuji apple, cored and chopped	*5* Pour the mayonnaise mix over the broccoli mix. Salt and pepper to taste and toss well.
¼ cup dried cranberries (no added sugar)	
Salt and ground black pepper to taste	*6* Add the chicken and toss again.
	7 Refrigerate at least 30 minutes and serve cold.

Per serving: *Kilojoules 1100/Calories 263 (From Fat 18); Fat 8g (Saturated 1.5g); Cholesterol 16mg; Sodium 147mg; Carbohydrate 8g (Dietary Fibre 2g); Protein 4g; Sugar 12.6g.*

Vary It! Sauté the chicken in ½ teaspoon of curry powder.

Vary It! For a less-crunchy variation, use steamed broccoli instead of raw.

Tip: Remove the cranberries from the recipe to lower the sugar content.

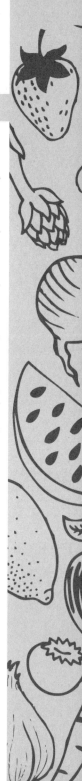

Almond Chicken Salad

Prep time: 5 min • **Yield:** 4 servings

Ingredients	Directions
2 cooked boneless, skinless chicken breasts (about 290 grams combined)	*1* Chop the cooked chicken breasts into bite-sized pieces.
⅓ cup almond slivers	*2* In a large bowl, mix the chicken, almonds, onion, celery, tarragon and mayonnaise. Salt and pepper to taste.
1 tablespoon chopped red onion	
1 tablespoon chopped celery	*3* Halve the lime and squeeze in lime juice. Mix thoroughly.
½ teaspoon tarragon	
½ cup whole egg mayonnaise	*4* Refrigerate or serve immediately on pita bread, flat bread or grain crackers.
1 fresh lime	
Salt and ground black pepper to taste	
4 pita halves or flat bread or grain crackers	

Per serving: Kilojoules 1218/Calories 291 (From Fat 156); Fat 17.4g (Saturated 2.7g); Cholesterol 67mg; Sodium 306mg; Carbohydrate 15.7g (Dietary Fibre 2g); Protein 25.6g; Sugar 3.3g.

Vary It! Use walnuts or pistachios instead of almonds.

Vary It! Serve the salad on a bed of mixed greens (such as spinach, rocket or romaine) instead of the pita bread, flat bread or crackers.

Greek Salad with Lamb

Prep time: 10 min • **Cook time:** 12 min • **Yield:** 4 servings

Ingredients	*Directions*
Olive oil (for coating fry pan) ½ kilogram of minced lamb (ask your butcher or slice a lamb backstrap)	*1* Very lightly coat a large fry pan with olive oil and heat it on medium heat.
Salt and ground black pepper to taste	*2* Brown the lamb in the fry pan, breaking it up as it cooks, for about 8 to 12 minutes. Remove from heat and drain off excess oil. Add salt and pepper to taste.
4 cups mixed green leaves	
1 cup cherry tomatoes	*3* In a large bowl, combine the greens, tomatoes, cucumber, olives, feta, oregano and lemon juice. Add the olive oil and vinegar, and salt and pepper to taste. Mix well.
1 medium cucumber, washed and sliced	
1 cup kalamata olives	
1 cup feta cheese	*4* Split the salad mix into four plates and divide the lamb among the plates. Add a few slices of red onion on top and serve.
1 teaspoon chopped fresh oregano	
1 tablespoon fresh lemon juice	
2 teaspoons cold-pressed or extra-virgin olive oil	
1 to 2 teaspoons red wine vinegar, to taste	
½ red onion	

Per serving: Kilojoules 1895/Calories 453 (From Fat 268); Fat 29.8g (Saturated 14.6g); Cholesterol 115mg; Sodium 782mg; Carbohydrate 11.3g (Dietary Fibre 3.2g); Protein 31.6g; Sugar 5.5g.

Vary It! For a vegetarian option, substitute 2 cups of chickpeas (drained and rinsed) for the minced lamb and mix through at Step 3.

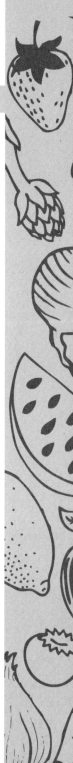

Vegetarian Wraps

Prep time: 10 min • **Cook time:** 10 min • **Yield:** 2 wraps

Ingredients	Directions
2 cups chopped mushrooms 2 teaspoons cold-pressed or extra-virgin olive oil	**1** In a medium fry pan, sauté the mushrooms in olive oil over medium-high heat. After 2 minutes, add the capsicum and continue cooking, stirring often.
1 medium red capsicum, sliced thinly 1 cup cooked chickpeas or kidney beans	**2** After about 3 to 5 more minutes, when the capsicum starts to soften, add the beans to the skillet to warm them for 3 to 4 more minutes. Stir often.
½ fresh lemon Salt and ground black pepper to taste 2 large whole-wheat tortillas	**3** When the pan veggies are fully cooked (about 10 minutes total), remove the pan from the heat. Squeeze lemon juice over the veggies. Add salt and pepper to taste.
2 cups fresh spinach or mixed green leaves ¼ avocado, chopped 1 medium tomato, chopped	**4** Microwave the tortillas for a few seconds to make them easier to wrap and less likely to break. Lay the warm tortillas flat and cover the centre with the greens, avocado and tomato.
	5 Top the tortillas with the warm veggie mix. Wrap them carefully and serve.

Per serving: Kilojoules 2046/Calories 489 (From Fat 138); Fat 15.4g (Saturated 4.4g); Cholesterol 0mg; Sodium 1052mg; Carbohydrate 72.2g (Dietary Fibre 12.7g); Protein 16.3g; Sugar 9.7g.

Crunchy Quinoa Cakes

Prep time: 15 min, plus refrigeration time • **Cook time:** 25 min • **Yield:** 4–6 servings

Ingredients	*Directions*
3 eggs	*1* Preheat oven to 200 degrees Celsius.
½ tablespoon coconut flour	
3 tablespoons tahini, almond or peanut butter	*2* In a large mixing bowl mix the eggs, tahini (or almond or peanut butter), vinegar and quinoa until well combined.
1 tablespoon red or white wine vinegar	
3 cups cooked quinoa, rinsed well	
¼ cup finely diced onion	*3* Add all remaining ingredients to the quinoa mix except the oil. Stir until everything is well combined. Let the mixture chill in the fridge for about 30 minutes.
2 garlic cloves (Australian or local), minced	
1 cup finely grated sweet potato	
1 300-gram box frozen chopped spinach, thawed and squeezed dry	*4* Make the quinoa cakes by placing 3 to 4 tablespoons of the mixture into your wet hands and firmly forming it into a round flat patty. Place the patty onto a well-oiled baking sheet. Bake, flipping halfway through, until lightly browned and just crisp, for about 25 minutes.
½ cup chopped nuts (pine nuts, walnuts or your very favourite nuts — optional)	
½ cup chopped sun-dried tomatoes	
¼ cup crumbled feta cheese	
2 tablespoons chopped parsley, dill or coriander	*5* Serve with tzatziki, chutney or tomato sauce.
1 teaspoon sea salt	
Black pepper, cumin and/or cayenne to taste	
Grape seed oil	
Tzatziki, chutney or tomato sauce (to serve)	

Per serving (based on 4 servings without sauce): Kilojoules 2114/Calories 505 (From Fat 207); Fat 23g (Saturated 4.8g); Cholesterol 147mg; Sodium 870mg; Carbohydrate 49.7g (Dietary Fibre 10.4g); Protein 20.5g; Sugar 3.3g.

Vary It! Use up your leftover veggies or add some frozen or fresh veggies and enjoy a nutritious meal.

Vary It! Add some lentils and curry powder at Step 3 to add an Indian taste. Or add a bunch of parsley at Step 3 and stuff patties into pita bread with lettuce and tahini sauce.

Source: Adapted from The Family Dinner recipe.

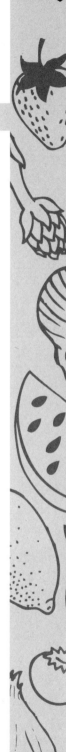

Mexican Rice

Prep time: 15 min • **Cook time:** Up to 60 min • **Yield:** 8 servings

Ingredients	Directions
4 cups MSG-free vegetable stock 2 cups brown rice	*1* In a medium pot, bring the vegetable stock to a boil. Add the rice, cover and simmer on low heat, stirring frequently.
1½ cups canned kidney beans	*2* Drain and rinse the beans to remove excess salt.
1 large tomato 2 large carrots 2 stalks celery	*3* Chop the tomato, carrots and celery so that they're all the same size.
Olive oil 1 cup diced red onion 1 tablespoon ground cumin 1 tablespoon ground coriander 2 teaspoons chilli powder	*4* Coat a medium saucepan in olive oil and combine the onion, carrots, celery, cumin, coriander and chilli powder. Cook 3 to 5 minutes over medium heat, stirring constantly, until the ingredients are browned. Add this into the simmering rice pot.
½ cup fresh or frozen corn kernels Garnish: Chopped fresh parsley and/or chopped fresh coriander	*5* After approximately 15 minutes, add the beans, chopped tomato and corn to the rice pot. Continue simmering while covered and continue to stir frequently. Cook the mixture until the stock is absorbed and the rice is fluffy (total cook time varies depending on rice variety).
	6 Remove from heat. Fluff the rice mixture with a fork, top with a sprinkling of parsley and/or coriander, and serve warm.

Per serving: Kilojoules 661/Calories 158 (From Fat 25); Fat 3g (Saturated 0.5g); Cholesterol 0mg; Sodium 666mg; Carbohydrate 29g (Dietary Fibre 6g); Protein 5g; Sugar 5.6g.

Vary It! For more protein, add some diced nitrate-free bacon to the vegetables in Step 4.

No Bread Beef Burgers

Prep time: 10 min • **Cook time:** 12 min • **Yield:** 4 servings

Ingredients	Directions
500 grams minced grass-fed beef **½ cup seasoned panko or Italian bread crumbs or gluten-free bread crumbs** **½ cup diced portobello mushroom** **2 tablespoons diced green capsicum** **1 tablespoon Worcestershire sauce** **½ cup grated Parmigiano cheese** **1 teaspoon olive oil** **1 head organic lettuce** **Salt and ground black pepper to taste**	**1** In a large bowl, combine the beef, bread crumbs, mushroom, capsicum, Worcestershire sauce and cheese. Mix thoroughly by hand. **2** Divide the meat mix into quarters to make four large burger patties approximately 1.5-centimetres thick. **3** Grease a grill or a fry pan with olive oil and cook the patties over medium heat, flipping once, until done to preference (5 or 6 minutes per side should do it). **4** Remove the patties and serve them wrapped in romaine lettuce leaves instead of on a traditional roll. (We recommend at least two pieces of lettuce for each 'slice' of roll on the top and bottom.) Add salt and pepper to taste.

Per serving: Kilojoules 1221/Calories 292 (From Fat 72); Fat 8g (Saturated 3.9g); Cholesterol 79mg; Sodium 579mg; Carbohydrate 16.2g (Dietary Fibre 2.6g); Protein 37.2g; Sugar 4.4g.

Vary It! For spicier burgers, add ½ teaspoon of chopped jalapeños or Cajun spice to Step 1. You can also top the burgers with the cheese of your choice.

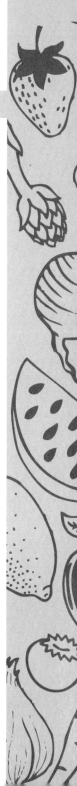

Red Lentil Soup

Prep time: 5 min • **Cook time:** 20 min • **Yield:** 5 servings

Ingredients	Directions
500 grams red lentils	**1** Rinse the lentils.
1 carrot, peeled	
1 large sweet potato, peeled	**2** Chop the carrot, sweet potato and celery so they're all the same size.
2 sticks celery	
1 leek, sliced	**3** Put all ingredients in a large pot over a medium heat. Bring to the boil (watch that the soup doesn't boil over because lentils foam when boiling), turn heat to low and simmer for 20 minutes.
1 small red onion, diced	
½ chilli	
½ teaspoon cinnamon	**4** Remove from heat and allow to cool slightly before puréeing. We used a stick blender for speed and convenience, but you can also use a regular blender or food processor.
2 garlic cloves (Australian or local)	
1.5 litres MSG-free vegetable or chicken stock	

Per serving: Kilojoules 2067/Calories 494 (From Fat 49); Fat 5.5g (Saturated 1.4g); Cholesterol 9mg; Sodium 477mg; Carbohydrate 80g (Dietary Fibre 12.8g); Protein 32.9g; Sugar 9.4g.

Tip: For an Asian influence, add coconut milk, chilli and a lemongrass stick. Add coconut milk at end and bring back to heat, taking care not to boil, otherwise it will curdle. Remove lemongrass stick before puréeing.

Tip: For a lower sugar meal omit the carrots and only use ½ a sweet potato.

Chicken Tenderloins with Corn Relish

Prep time: 15 min • **Cook time:** 15 min • **Yield:** 4 servings

Ingredients	Directions
1 teaspoon plus 3 tablespoons olive oil, divided	*1* Grease an iron fry pan with 1 teaspoon of olive oil and heat over medium-high heat.
½ teaspoon paprika	
½ teaspoon dry mustard	*2* In a small bowl, mix 3 tablespoons olive oil, paprika, mustard, cayenne, salt and pepper. Remove 1 teaspoon of this seasoned oil to add to the corn relish.
¼ teaspoon cayenne pepper	
¼ teaspoon salt	
¼ teaspoon ground black pepper	*3* Brush the chicken heavily with the remaining seasoned oil.
Eight chicken tenderloins	*4* When the skillet is hot, sear the tenderloins for 2 minutes on one side. Turn them with tongs, cover and turn off the heat. Allow the tenderloins to rest in the skillet for 4 to 5 minutes.
Corn Relish (see the following recipe)	
	5 Serve the warm tenderloins topped with the cold Corn Relish.

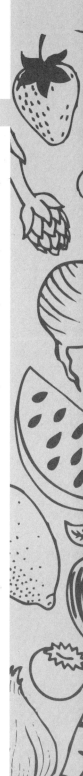

Corn Relish

1 cup frozen corn kernels
(about 2 ears if fresh)

¼ cup diced red capsicum

2 tablespoons chopped red
onion

2 tablespoons chopped white
onion

2 tablespoons chopped celery

¼ cup cider vinegar

1 tablespoon olive oil

Salt and ground black pepper
to taste

1 Cook frozen corn according to package instructions. If
you're using fresh corn, fill a small saucepan halfway
with salted water and bring it to a boil. Add the corn
and cook it for approximately 5 minutes, until the corn
is tender. Drain and cool the corn under cold running
water. Shake off excess water in a strainer. Pat the corn
kernels dry.

2 In a medium bowl, mix the corn, capsicum, red onion,
white onion, celery, vinegar and oil. Add the seasoned
oil mix that you set aside while preparing the chicken
tenderloins. Mix well and refrigerate.

Per serving: Kilojoules 1313/Calories 314 (From Fat 150); Fat 16.7g (Saturated 2.8g); Cholesterol 75mg;
Sodium 285mg; Carbohydrate 11.2g (Dietary Fibre 1.6g); Protein 26.7g; Sugar 1.6g.

Tip: Garnish the chicken tenderloins with dark greens like kale or flat leaf parsley for additional
iron.

Making smart lunch choices

If you eat a high-protein, fibre-filled lunch with
lots of organic vegetables, you'll likely stay satisfied, energised and craving-free for the rest
of the day.

Lunches that contain mostly high-glycaemic
carbs — lots of bread, pasta or sugar — lead to
a sleepy, brain-fogged afternoon. A high-insulin
afternoon makes you feel sluggish, increases
your fat storage and makes you crave carbs
later in the day. Cut back on lunchtime carbs
by choosing meals like a mixed green salad

with grilled chicken instead of a chicken pasta
dish. Using lettuce or kale as the top piece of
sandwich bread halves the amount of bread
and gives you extra leafy greens to boot.
Sometimes, Michele just uses lettuce to make
her sandwich. Sounds strange, but try it.

Use lunch as an opportunity to increase the
amount of vegetables in your diet. Load up your
sandwich with extra spinach, rocket, tomato,
onion, capsicum, olives, mushrooms, or whatever other veggies you like.

Chapter 15

Nourishing, Easy Dinners

In This Chapter

▶ Making healthy dinners quickly

▶ Checking out some speedy dinner recipes

*W*e'd like to emphasise the 'easy' part in the title of this chapter. Cooking a healthy dinner doesn't have to be stressful — in fact, it could be the most de-stressing part of your day. Making dinnertime stress-free takes time and planning in the beginning, but gets easier with a well-stocked pantry and refrigerator. In this chapter, we take you through some quick and nourishing options to get you started.

Dinnertime isn't just about the food; the time should be nourishing on all levels. The evening family meal is becoming a lost tradition, but it may be the only time a family connects during the day. If the tradition has been lost in your family, try to reinstate it. Not only does sharing the meal together prevent you and your family from mindless eating in front of the television, but it also allows you the opportunity to listen, learn and bond.

Creating Fast and Nourishing Dinners

One difficulty that lots of clients have expressed to us over the years is finding the time to cook healthy meals. When you work long days and the kids have after-school activities, you don't have a lot of time left for cooking. Here are some tips for cutting down your time in the kitchen:

✔ **Build a repertoire of dependable recipes.** Master a handful of recipes so you can make them without thinking. That way you always have a healthy fallback if you're pressed for time when 6 pm rolls around.

✔ **Plan your menus several days ahead.** That way you have plenty of time to procure any special ingredients, and when it's time to hit the kitchen, you already know what's going to happen and you're ready to dive in.

✔ **Read through the recipe first.** Before you start cooking, make sure you have all the ingredients on hand. To speed the process, look for places you can multi-task — for example, while water is boiling or food is cooking.

✔ **Make a list and do a major shop one day per week.** Walking aimlessly around the shops is a waste of time. If you have planned your menu, read the recipe, make a list and head for the shops. Shopping in the early morning hours on a Saturday or Sunday is a good option because the stores are usually quiet and you can move through quickly.

✔ **Do the prep for several meals at once.** Plan your meals for a few days at a time and, when you're chopping up stuff for one of them, do the prep work for the next meal or two while you have the cutting board out. Fill storage containers with ingredients ready to grab for the next few times you're cooking.

✔ **Enjoy the process.** Find pleasure in the process of preparing healthy food for your family. They may enjoy getting involved too! You may be surprised how much you can find out about your child's or partner's day while they are cutting vegetables and you are marinating meat!

✔ **Find some organic, low-sugar bottled sauces.** Premade sauces can add some zing to an otherwise uninspiring chicken-and-veggie dish. Experiment with prepared salsa, teriyaki, hoisin or pesto sauces — the low-sugar kinds, of course!

Food needs to taste good for you to be able to sustain a low-sugar way of life. Marinate your quality proteins in sauces and spices and garnish with pesto so that your variety of foods seems more expansive than it actually is. Grilled Indian chicken breast, for example, can taste very different from Green Chicken Curry, but it is still quality chicken protein — just with a different sauce. Some sauces that are low-sugar and free of preservatives, additives or colours include tamari (a wheat-free soy sauce) and Bragg Liquid Aminos (a liquid protein concentrate, derived from soybeans). (See www.ahealthyview.com.au for more options.)

You can make double quantities for most of the recipes in this chapter to follow the 'cook once, eat twice' rule — that is, create leftovers for lunches and other meals — and make your meals easier.

How to thaw meat quickly

The best way to thaw frozen meat is not to leave it thawing in the sink but to move it to the refrigerator, where it will thaw evenly in a day or two and stay at a safe temperature the whole time. However, sometimes forgetfulness or a last-minute change of plans requires you to cook something that's still frozen.

Don't defrost meat in the microwave. It heats too unevenly, and you'll have some parts partially cooked and some parts still frozen. The meat then won't cook well in the oven or on the stovetop.

Don't run a package of meat under hot (or even warm) water. Doing so starts to cook the meat on the outer edges.

The correct way to thaw frozen meat quickly is to place the package in a bowl filled with cold water and place the bowl under the kitchen tap with a cold-water drip. Adjust the tap so you get a tiny stream of water, just slightly faster than being able to count the drips. Rotate the package occasionally.

Lemon Caper Blue Eye Trevalla

Prep time: 6 min • **Cook time:** 10–15 min • **Yield:** 4 servings

Ingredients	Directions
3 tablespoons olive oil, divided	**1** Heat 1 tablespoon of olive oil in a small saucepan over medium heat. When the oil is hot, sauté the shallots for about 1½ minutes.
1 shallot, minced	
½ cup white wine	**2** Add the wine and increase the heat to high. Boil 3 to 5 minutes, until the sauce is reduced to approximately ¼ cup.
2 tablespoons butter	
1 tablespoon chopped fresh flat-leaf parsley	**3** Strain the sauce and discard the shallot pieces. Return the sauce to the pan over medium heat.
Juice of ½ lemon	
¼ cup rice flour	**4** Add the butter and parsley and whisk to combine. Add the lemon juice to the mixture and stir briefly (watch out for lemon seeds). Set the sauce aside.
Sprinkle of salt and ground black pepper	
4 large blue eyed cod fillets (or barramundi or any white fish fillet)	**5** Heat the remaining 2 tablespoons of olive oil in a large fry pan on medium-high heat until it's simmering but not smoking. If the oil smokes, it's too hot and you need to start over with fresh oil.
2 tablespoons capers	
	6 While the oil heats, spread the rice flour on a plate and sprinkle it with salt and pepper.
	7 Rinse the fish fillets in cold water, and then coat both sides of each fillet in the rice flour mix.
	8 When the oil is heated, place the fillets in the fry pan and reduce to medium heat.

9 Cook the fillets for 2 to 3 minutes on one side, until the edges are opaque and the bottoms are browned.

10 Flip the fillets and sprinkle the capers on top. Cook on this side for 2 to 3 minutes, until the bottom is brown and the thickest part of the fillet is soft.

11 Plate each fillet and top with the desired amount of sauce. Be sure to get some capers onto each fillet.

Per serving: Kilojoules 1523/Calories 364 (From Fat 144); Fat 16.1g (Saturated 5.3g); Cholesterol 124mg; Sodium 832mg; Carbohydrate 9.8g (Dietary Fibre 0.4g); Protein 36.3g; Sugar 0.5g.

Tip: Serve fish fillets over a bed of fresh spinach sautéed in olive oil and garnished with fresh lemon rind.

Looking at wild-caught versus farmed salmon

Eating fish is good for your health, but when it comes to what sort of fish you should eat, you're faced with some choices — for example, what has the highest nutrient density versus what is ethical and sustainable? Farmed salmon can result in a drop in omega-3 levels but the Aquaculture Stewardship Council argues that this type of farmed fish still remains a good choice for these healthy fats.

We suggest choosing wild-caught salmon if you can find it. If you can't find wild-caught, ask your fishmonger what type of food was fed to the fish, and what kind of practices the producers follow. For example, Tassal, which farms Atlantic salmon in Tasmania, uses feed with a percentage of vegetable and poultry meal (substituted for wild fish ingredients) that meets Aquaculture Stewardship Council standards for sustainable seafood. The company is also introducing better netting so they catch only what they intend to, and protect other wildlife. Tassal also monitors the levels of organic waste flowing into nearby waters and keeps them low.

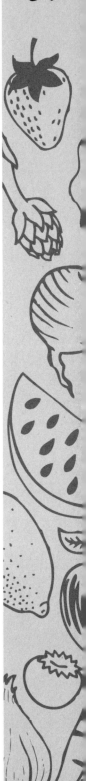

Grilled Salmon with Coriander Salsa

Prep time: 10 min • **Cook time:** 15–20 min • **Yield:** 6 servings

Ingredients	Directions
1 kilogram wild-caught salmon 1 tablespoon extra-virgin olive oil 1 pinch sea salt 1 pinch black pepper 1 small bunch coriander, including stems, rinsed 2 tablespoons fresh mint leaves, chopped 3 tablespoons extra-virgin olive oil (for salsa) 1½ tablespoons garlic, minced 1 pinch sea salt 1 tablespoon fresh lemon or lime juice 1 pinch chilli pepper flakes (optional)	**1** Season salmon with olive oil, salt and pepper. Set aside for 10 minutes. **2** For salsa, combine all remaining ingredients in a blender. Blend until smooth and fragrant. Set aside. **3** Heat a griddle, grill or fry pan on medium-high heat and place fish on grill, skin side down. Allow salmon to cook until skin is charred and fish is almost cooked through. This will take about 15 minutes, depending on the thickness of the salmon. **4** Turn salmon over and grill a few more minutes, until fish is fully cooked. **5** Remove salmon from heat and lay skin side up on a platter. Pull skin off salmon (if preferred) and flip back to serve. **6** Spread salsa on top of salmon. Serve with wedges of lemon or lime.

Per serving: Kilojoules 1473/Calories 352 (From Fat 154); Fat 17.2g (Saturated 2.9g); Cholesterol 106mg; Sodium 295mg; Carbohydrate 3.8g (Dietary Fibre 2.2g); Protein 37.3g; Sugar 0.06g.

Tip: Serve with a side of steamed asparagus or sautéed spinach.

Too Easy Salmon Cakes

Prep time: 5 min • **Cook time:** 10 min • **Yield:** 6 servings

Ingredients	*Directions*
425-gram can boneless salmon	*1* Mix salmon with onion, celery, dill, lemon juice and salt.
1 white onion, diced	
2 celery stalks, sliced	*2* Add coconut flour and combine thoroughly.
2 tablespoons fresh finely chopped dill	*3* Add eggs in and mix until well combined.
2 teaspoons lemon juice	
½ teaspoon sea salt	*4* Warm fry pan over medium heat and melt coconut oil.
2½ tablespoons coconut flour	*5* Form salmon mix into patties and place on pan to cook.
4 free-range eggs	
6 tablespoons extra-virgin coconut oil	*6* Cook until brown on both sides, approximately 4 minutes each side.

Per serving: Kilojoules 1276/Calories 305 (From Fat 179); Fat 19.9g (Saturated 14.1g); Cholesterol 155mg; Sodium 513mg; Carbohydrate 4.8g (Dietary Fibre 1.9g); Protein 21.5g; Sugar 1.3g.

Vary It! Use canned tuna instead of salmon.

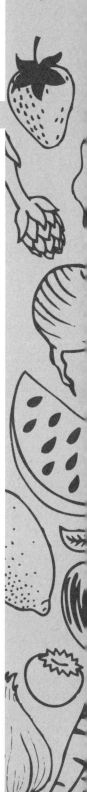

Coconut Lime Prawns

Prep time: 8 min • **Cook time:** 35 min • **Yield:** 4 servings

Ingredients	Directions
MSG-free vegetable (or chicken or fish) stock	**1** Boil a mixture of half stock and half water and cook the rice or quinoa according to the package instructions. (Using vegetable, chicken or fish stock with the water adds additional flavour.)
1 cup basmati rice or quinoa	
1 lime	**2** Zest a small amount of lime on a cheese grater.
½ kilogram fresh Australian (or local) uncooked prawns, peeled and deveined	**3** In a bowl, add the prawns, lime zest and a pinch of salt. Squeeze in the lime juice and let marinate for 15 minutes.
Sea salt	
2 teaspoons olive oil	**4** In a large fry pan, heat the olive oil over medium heat. Sauté the prawns for 1 to 2 minutes and then remove them from the pan and set aside.
¾ cup unsweetened coconut milk	
¼ cup chopped fresh coriander	**5** In the same pan, combine the coconut milk, coriander, mint, spring onions and peanuts. Cook for 1 minute.
2 tablespoons chopped mint	
4 spring onions (both white and green parts), chopped	
2 tablespoons chopped unsalted roasted peanuts	**6** Stir in the prawns and cook for 1 minute more, stirring constantly.
	7 Serve the prawns and sauce on a bed of rice or quinoa.

Per serving: Kilojoules 1677/Calories 401 (From Fat 148); Fat 16g (Saturated 10g); Cholesterol 143mg; Sodium 352mg; Carbohydrate 44g (Dietary Fibre 2.5g); Protein 21g; Sugar 1.06.

Tip: To add some zing, add a chopped Thai chilli.

Lean Beef Stir-Fry

Prep time: 15 min • **Cook time:** 10 min • **Yield:** 8 servings

Ingredients	Directions
4 teaspoons coconut oil, butter or ghee	**1** Heat the oil in the wok and brown the beef in batches for about 2 minutes. Remove from heat.
800 grams scotch or rump beef, sliced thinly	
10 green onions, cut into lengths about 6-centimetres long	**2** Place the green onions, broccolini, snow peas and chilli in a bowl and sprinkle the sesame oil over them.
12 broccolini spears, trimmed and cut in half	**3** Add the vegetable mix to the wok and cook for 2 to 3 minutes. Stir through the ginger, tamari, mirin, sake and cooked beef and stir until heated through.
2 cups snow peas	
1 chilli (optional)	
2 teaspoons toasted sesame oil	**4** Sprinkle the sesame seeds through and serve.
2 teaspoons chopped ginger	
½ cup wheat-free soy tamari	
½ cup mirin	
2 tablespoons sake	
4 tablespoons sesame seeds	

Per serving: Kilojoules 1326/Calories 317 (From Fat 149); Fat 16.6g (Saturated 7.0g); Cholesterol 84mg; Sodium 1069mg; Carbohydrate 6.6g (Dietary Fibre 2.6g); Protein 30.2g; Sugar 1.8g.

Vary It! Experiment with different kinds of seafood instead of the beef, such as prawns or tuna.

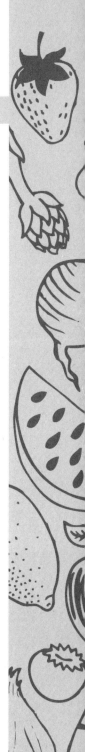

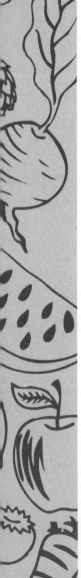

Chilli Chicken Tenderloins

Prep time: 20 min • **Cook time:** 15 min • **Yield:** 4 servings

Ingredients	Directions
500 grams chicken tenderloins	**1** Preheat the oven to 180 degrees Celsius.
1 tablespoon local honey	
2 tablespoons butter	**2** Flatten chicken tenderloins with a meat mallet until they're ½-centimetre thick.
¼ teaspoon chilli flakes (or more to taste)	**3** In a small saucepan, warm the honey on medium-low heat, taking care not to boil it. Add the butter and stir.
½ teaspoon paprika	
Salt	**4** When the butter has melted, remove from the heat and stir in the chilli flakes, paprika and a pinch of salt.
2 cups cubed sweet potatoes	
1 teaspoon fresh rosemary	**5** Spread the sweet potato on a large baking sheet drizzled with olive oil. Sprinkle with rosemary, salt and pepper. Roast for approximately 10 minutes, until the potatoes are tender.
Sprinkle of ground black pepper	
2 tablespoons olive oil	**6** While the potatoes are roasting, coat a large fry pan with 1 tablespoon olive oil and heat over medium heat. Sauté the chicken for 2 to 3 minutes on one side, until golden-brown. Flip the chicken.
	7 Add the honey chilli sauce to the pan with the chicken and cook for 2 to 3 minutes, until the chicken is cooked and the sauce is slightly thick.
	8 Place chicken on a dinner plate and top with about a tablespoon of chilli sauce for each serve. Serve with ½ cup of sweet potato drizzled with 1 tablespoon olive oil.

Per serving: Kilojoules 1364/Calories 326 (From Fat 127); Fat 14.2g (Saturated 5.3g); Cholesterol 95mg; Sodium 181mg; Carbohydrate 18.1g (Dietary Fibre 2.3g); Protein 27.7g; Sugar 7.1g.

Tip: Serve with a side of steamed broccoli or a large, mixed green salad.

Baked Parmesan Chicken

Prep time: 7 min • **Cook time:** 40–50 min • **Yield:** 4 servings

Ingredients	Directions
4 boneless, skinless chicken breasts	*1* Preheat the oven to 180 degrees Celsius. Grease a baking dish with butter.
½ cup Italian or gluten-free bread crumbs	*2* Rinse the chicken breasts under cold tap water and set them aside.
½ cup freshly grated parmigiano cheese	*3* Mix the bread crumbs, cheese, Fresh Italian Seasoning, salt and pepper in a shallow dish.
¼ cup Fresh Italian Seasoning (see the following recipe)	*4* Beat the egg in a separate shallow dish.
½ teaspoon salt	*5* Dip each chicken breast in the egg and then press it into the seasoned crumb mix, coating both sides heavily. Place in the baking dish.
¼ teaspoon ground black pepper	
1 large egg	*6* Bake chicken breasts uncovered for 40 to 50 minutes, until chicken is cooked through.

Fresh Italian Seasoning

2 tablespoons minced fresh basil	*1* Mix all ingredients together in a small bowl.
1 tablespoon minced fresh oregano	
2 tablespoons minced fresh parsley	
2 Australian (or local) garlic cloves, minced	

Per serving: Kilojoules 1175/Calories 281 (From Fat 80); Fat 9g (Saturated 3.5g); Cholesterol 150mg; Sodium 482mg; Carbohydrate 6g (Dietary Fibre 1g); Protein 42g; Sugar 1.05g.

Tip: Because the bake time on this dish is almost an hour, it may work better as a weekend dinner or when you're not rushed for time.

Tip: This dish goes well with sweet potato mash. It's also excellent with a strong-flavoured green like kale or a rocket salad.

Grilled Cajun Beef Kebabs

Prep time: 12 min • **Cook time:** 8–9 min • **Yield:** 8 servings

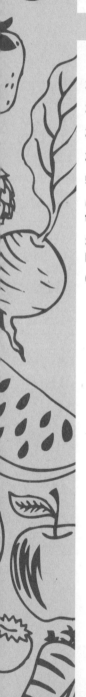

Ingredients	Directions
16 wooden skewers	*1* Soak the wooden skewers in warm water for 20 to 30 minutes. Preheat a charcoal or gas grill.
2 large green capsicums	
24 cherry tomatoes	*2* Wash all the vegetables and cut everything except the cherry tomatoes into squares approximately 2×2 centimetre.
2 red onions	
2 large mushrooms	
500 grams beef fillet	*3* Cut the beef into 2-centimetre cubes and dip them into the Cajun Basting Sauce.
Cajun Basting Sauce (see the following recipe)	
Salt and ground black pepper	*4* Alternate skewering pieces of capsicum, tomato, beef, onion and mushroom onto skewers until they're full.
Olive oil (for cooking)	
	5 Heavily brush the kebabs with the Cajun Basting Sauce. Sprinkle the kebabs with salt and pepper.
	6 Brush the grill with olive oil. Grill the kebabs with the grill lid closed, until the edges of the meat and vegetables are crispy (approximately 8 to 9 minutes), using tongs to turn the skewers frequently.

Cajun Basting Sauce

¼ cup olive oil

Juice of 1 lime

1 teaspoon minced fresh oregano

2 tablespoons Cajun spice

1 teaspoon Worcestershire sauce

1 Whisk together all ingredients in a small bowl.

Per serving: Kilojoules 1121/Calories 268 (From Fat 149); Fat 16.6g (Saturated 5.5g); Cholesterol 53mg; Sodium 50mg; Carbohydrate 12.7g (Dietary Fibre 2.9g); Protein 14.6g; Sugar 6.9g.

Tip: Cajun spice mix is available from most supermarkets, but you can get some excellent spices online — try www.thespicetradingcompany.com.au.

Vary It! Serve mini-kebabs as an appetiser or use them as a snack to take to work. On a short skewer, slide one piece of beef in between two vegetables.

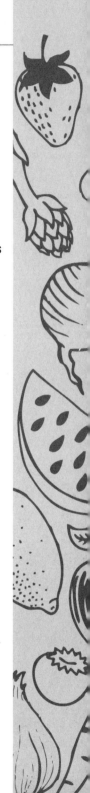

Lamb Wraps

Prep time: 25 min, plus refrigeration time • **Cook time:** 12 min • **Yield:** 4–6 pockets

Ingredients	Directions
500 grams minced lamb	*1* Brown the minced lamb in a fry pan over medium heat, stirring often. Don't overcook. Add spices to taste.
2 teaspoons red curry powder or ground cumin	
2 tablespoons minced red onion	*2* When the lamb is approximately halfway cooked (about 4 minutes), sprinkle the red onion into the pan.
4 whole-wheat tortilla or flat bread	*3* Warm the bread. Stir the refrigerated Tzatziki Sauce with a spoon and spread over the bread.
Tzatziki Sauce (see the following recipe)	
Handful of fresh lettuce	*4* Lay fresh lettuce and spinach to taste over the bread.
Handful of fresh spinach	*5* When the lamb is fully cooked, scoop a half-cup serving into a separate bowl. Add a teaspoon (or more, if you like) of Tzatziki Sauce and mix.
	6 Spread the sauced lamb onto the tortilla or flat bread and roll up. Enjoy hot.

Tzatziki Sauce

2 medium cucumbers

½ teaspoon sea salt

1 small clove garlic, minced

Juice of 1 lemon

Ground black pepper

3 cups plain Greek yoghurt

1 tablespoon chopped
fresh dill

1 Peel the cucumbers and cut them in half lengthwise. Scoop out the seeds with a spoon.

2 Dice the cucumbers and press them dry with a paper towel. Sprinkle with salt.

3 Place the salted cucumber, garlic, lemon juice and a few grinds of black pepper in a blender or food processor and process on medium speed until well blended.

4 Stir this mix into the Greek yoghurt. Add the dill and stir thoroughly. Refrigerate, preferably for several hours to allow the flavours to blend. You'll need to re-stir the sauce every time you use it.

Per serving: Kilojoules 1960/Calories 478 (From Fat 205); Fat 23g (Saturated 10g); Cholesterol 66mg; Sodium 730mg; Carbohydrate 35g (Dietary Fibre 5g); Protein 34g; Sugar 2.7g.

Tip: Although the hot lamb contrasted with the cold cucumber is appealing to some, you may want to place the assembled wrap in a sandwich press for 30 seconds if you prefer it warm.

Tip: If you double or triple the Tzatziki Sauce recipe, you can use it the next day as a dip with fresh, raw vegetables and/or on a tuna salad.

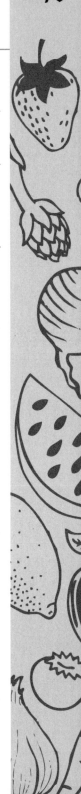

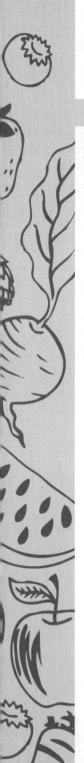

Vegetarian Pasta Pomodoro

Prep time: 8 min • **Cook time:** 25 min • **Yield:** 4 servings

Ingredients	Directions
Pomodoro Sauce (see the following recipe)	*1* Prepare the Pomodoro Sauce.
Sea salt	*2* While the sauce is simmering, boil 5 to 6 cups of salted water in a large saucepan. While the water is heating, wash and chop the zucchini, squash and mushrooms.
5–6 cups water	
1 small zucchini	
1 small yellow squash	*3* Add the pasta to the boiling water and cook according to label (approximately 8 minutes), stirring occasionally.
½ cup chopped mushrooms of your choice	
8 ounces brown rice pasta or gluten-free pasta	*4* While the pasta cooks, sauté the zucchini, squash and mushrooms in a small saucepan with olive oil.
2 tablespoons olive oil	
	5 Drain pasta and serve it topped with vegetables and Pomodoro Sauce.

Pomodoro Sauce

1 carrot	**1** Dice the carrot and celery, and mince the garlic.
1 celery stalk	
1 clove garlic	**2** Lightly coat a medium sauté pan with olive oil, and sauté the carrot, celery and garlic over medium heat until golden. Add salt.
¼ teaspoon salt	
425-millilitre can diced organic tomatoes	**3** Add the diced tomatoes, olive oil, bay leaf and vegetable broth (or stock). Stir in the tomato paste.
2 tablespoons extra-virgin or cold-pressed olive oil	
1 bay leaf	**4** Simmer (barely) for 15 to 20 minutes, stirring occasionally. Do not boil!
¼ cup vegetable broth or stock	
½ cup tomato paste	**5** Before serving, remove the bay leaf. Sprinkle with basil and oregano when serving.
1 tablespoon chopped fresh basil	
1 teaspoon chopped fresh oregano	

Per serving: Kilojoules 1267/Calories 303 (From Fat 101); Fat 11g (Saturated 2.5g); Cholesterol 19mg; Sodium 1383mg; Carbohydrate 28g (Dietary Fibre 4.5g); Protein 7g; Sugar 7.4g.

Vary It! Combine pasta with a piece of grilled fish or chicken, or add a cup of chickpeas to the pasta to increase the protein component.

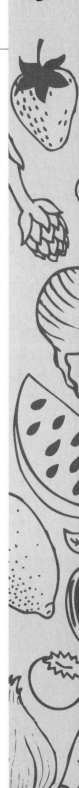

Vegetarian Chilli Goodness

Prep time: 8 min • **Cook time:** 1–2 hours • **Yield:** 8–10 servings

Ingredients	Directions

Ingredients

⅓ cup olive oil

1 large red onion, peeled, finely chopped

1 small red chilli, seeded, chopped

½ red capsicum, chopped

½ green capsicum, chopped

¼ teaspoon chilli flakes

½ teaspoon smoked paprika

½ teaspoon ground cinnamon

1 teaspoon ground cumin

1 teaspoon dried thyme

2 to 3 Australian (or local) garlic cloves, crushed

425-gram can organic kidney beans, drained, rinsed

425-gram can organic lentils, drained, rinsed

425-gram can diced tomatoes

1 tablespoon tomato paste

1 cup chopped flat-leaf parsley

Directions

1 Place 2 tablespoons of the olive oil in a large saucepan over medium heat. Add the onion, fresh chilli and capsicum and cook until softened.

2 Add the chilli flakes, paprika, cinnamon, cumin and thyme and cook for a further minute.

3 Reduce heat to low and add the garlic, beans, lentils, tomatoes, tomato paste and remaining oil.

4 Cover and simmer for 15 minutes, stirring occasionally.

5 Remove lid and cook for a further 5 minutes or until thickened.

6 Stir through the parsley and serve with steamed brown rice and sprinkled with grated cheese, if desired.

Per serving (based on 8 serves): Kilojoules 887/Calories 212 (From Fat 86); Fat 9.6g (Saturated 1.4g); Cholesterol 0mg; Sodium 363mg; Carbohydrate 24.2g (Dietary Fibre 8.6g); Protein 8.8g; Sugar 4.4g.

Vary It! Spoon chilli into hot flour tortillas along with condiments such as sour cream, shredded cheese and avocado for burrito filling.

Chapter 16

Satisfying Snacks

In This Chapter

▶ Choosing snacks that add nutrition to your diet

▶ Whipping up some healthy and delicious snacks

*H*ealthy snacks are crucial for keeping your blood sugar levels steady and for fending off sugar cravings. The right snacks satisfy your hunger and fuel your body for a few hours, leaving you sharp, energetic and craving-free. The wrong snacks (or no snacks at all) cause that familiar midafternoon sinking feeling and fog, which triggers a drive for something sweet.

Many of the snack recipes in this chapter are designed to be prepared and portioned out in advance so that they're easy to grab when you need a healthy snack in a hurry. You can find a high-protein apple walnut loaf, nutritious veggie burgers, spicy nuts, quiche muffins and delicious protein bars that will be ready to go when you are!

Understanding Snacking Success

When planning your snacks, think of them as mini-meals. Eating a protein-based snack ensures your blood sugar levels stay at a stable level for sustained energy and a feeling of satisfaction.

Healthy snacks add quality nutrition to your daily diet. Use your prepared snacks as an opportunity to put more vitamins, minerals, protein and antioxidants into your body. Grabbing something from a vending machine or from the lolly dish just adds extra calories without any worthwhile nutrients.

TIP

Plan ahead! If you leave the house without knowing what you're going to eat throughout the day, you leave yourself at the mercy of whatever is lying around in the break room at work, or whatever you can grab at a convenience store or drive-through fast food restaurant. Be smart and purposeful in your food planning so you can avoid reactive eating and stay a step ahead of those wicked sugar cravings!

Need a snack in a pinch? Eggs to the rescue!

A hard-boiled egg can be your go-to snack if you have zero time to get something healthy to eat. Downing an egg or two quells your hunger, adds extra protein for the day, and keeps your starving brain from driving you to sugar.

A common problem with hard-boiling eggs is that you can easily overcook them, leading to a dark green tint around the yolk and a sulphur taste. To boil eggs without overcooking, place a dozen pasture-fed eggs in a saucepan and add cold water until the top of the water line is 4 centimetres above the eggs. To keep the eggs from cracking, salt the water and gradually bring it to a boil. When the water is boiling, reduce the heat and simmer for about a minute. Then remove the pan from the burner, cover, and let sit for 12 minutes. Extra-large eggs need a few minutes more (15 to 17 minutes). If you're

cooking half a dozen eggs, you can cut the time to 9 minutes.

Remove the eggs with a slotted spoon and place them into a bowl of ice water. After they cool, strain the water from the eggs and refrigerate them in a covered container to protect your refrigerator from a strong egg odour. Eggs that have been refrigerated for a few days peel easier than fresher eggs.

One way to test whether your eggs are fully cooked is to set the larger end of the boiled egg on a hard surface, like a countertop or a table. Spin the egg the same way you would spin a top. A hard-boiled egg spins evenly and swiftly because the yolk is solid. An egg with an undercooked yolk doesn't spin well; it wobbles around instead of spinning in one spot.

Apple Cinnamon Walnut Loaf

Prep time: 10 min • **Cook time:** 50–60 min • **Yield:** 12 servings

Ingredients	Directions

Ingredients

3 tablespoons milk

6 tablespoons softened butter

2 tablespoons local honey

2 eggs

1 scoop (20 grams or
4 teaspoons) clean whey
protein powder (vanilla or
unflavoured)

1¾ cups plain unbleached
flour

1 teaspoon baking powder

½ teaspoon salt

½ teaspoon baking soda

1 cup unsweetened
applesauce

1 teaspoon ground cinnamon

170 grams walnuts, chopped

Directions

1 Preheat the oven to 175 degrees Celsius. Grease and flour a loaf tin.

2 Mix the milk, butter and honey in a medium bowl with an electric mixer on medium speed until the mix is light and fluffy. Gradually add the eggs and whey powder while continuing to beat.

3 In a separate bowl, mix together the flour, baking powder, salt and baking soda. Whisk this mix into the butter/egg batter until blended.

4 Stir in the applesauce, cinnamon and walnuts until blended.

5 Pour the batter into the loaf pan and bake for 50 to 60 minutes, until a toothpick inserted into the centre comes out clean.

6 Remove the loaf from the oven and cool it in the tin on a wire rack for 10 minutes. Remove the loaf from the tin and finish cooling it on the rack. Store at room temperature wrapped in foil.

Per serving: Kilojoules 1054/Calories 252 (From Fat 148); Fat 16g (Saturated 5g); Cholesterol 50mg; Sodium 454mg; Carbohydrate 21g (Dietary Fibre 2g); Protein 7g; Sugar 5.5g.

Vary It! For a completely gluten-free version, replace the flour with a half-and-half mix of quinoa and rice flour.

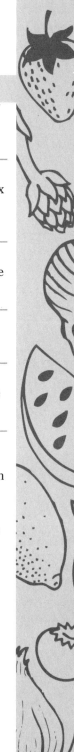

Chocolate Peanut Butter Protein Bars

Prep time: 10 min • **Cook time:** 5 min • **Yield:** 24 bars

Ingredients	*Directions*
1 cup creamy all-natural peanut butter	*1* In a glass bowl, stir together the peanut butter and honey. Microwave for 60 seconds, until the mixture stirs easily.
¼ cup local honey	
½ cup slow-cook oats	*2* In a separate bowl, blend together the oats, almond meal and cocoa powder.
¾ cup almond meal	
2 tablespoons cocoa powder	*3* Add the oats mix to the peanut butter and honey and mix thoroughly (it will be very thick).
85 grams dark chocolate (70% cocoa)	
	4 Press the mixture into a 22-×-40-centimetre baking tray, approximately 2 cm thick. As another option, you can roll the mixture into balls instead.
	5 Place the baking pan in the freezer for 5 to 10 minutes, until the mix starts to harden a little.
	6 In a medium saucepan, slowly melt the chocolate. When the chocolate is melted, remove the pan from the freezer and coat the mix with the melted chocolate.
	7 Return the pan to the freezer; remove it when the chocolate hardens.
	8 Cut into 24 servings. Serve at room temperature.

Per serving: *Kilojoules 623/Calories 149 (From Fat 84); Fat 9g (Saturated 2.5g); Cholesterol 17mg; Sodium 67mg; Carbohydrate 8g (Dietary Fibre 1.5g); Protein 10g; Sugar 4.9g.*

Vary It! Add ¼ cup coconut or pecan pieces to Step 2.

Vary It! Add 1 cup 'clean' whey protein powder (vanilla or unflavoured) in Step 2.

Three Bean Quinoa Salad

Prep time: 5 min • **Cook time:** 25 min • **Yield:** 6 servings

Ingredients	*Directions*
2 cups water	*1* In a medium saucepan, bring the water to a boil. Add the quinoa, cover and reduce the heat. Simmer for approximately 20 minutes, until the water is absorbed. Remove from the heat and fluff the quinoa with a fork.
1 cup quinoa	
425-gram can black beans, drained and rinsed	
425-gram can kidney beans, drained and rinsed	*2* Mix in the beans, olive oil, vinegar and Italian herbs. Stir well. Salt and pepper to taste.
425-gram can cannellini beans, drained and rinsed	
¼ cup extra-virgin olive oil	*3* Refrigerate for at least two hours before serving.
¼ cup red wine vinegar	
2 teaspoons dried Italian herbs	
Salt and ground black pepper to taste	

Per serving: Kilojoules 1238/Calories 296 (From Fat 90); Fat 10g (Saturated 1.5g); Cholesterol 0mg; Sodium 458mg; Carbohydrate 42g (Dietary Fibre 11g); Protein 13g; Sugar 1.4g.

Vary It! Add ½ cup chopped roasted red capsicum or chopped kalamata olives to Step 2.

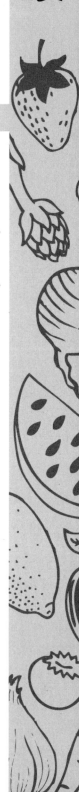

Chicken Nachos

Prep time: 5 min • **Cook time:** 15 min • **Yield:** 6–8 servings

Ingredients	Directions
225 grams ground chicken mince	**1** Coat a medium fry pan with a dash of olive oil. Combine the chicken mince, onion and capsicum in the pan. Cook over medium heat, stirring often, until the chicken mince is browned (about 7 minutes).
½ cup chopped onion	
½ cup chopped red capsicum	
½ cup chopped green or jalapeño pepper	**2** Stir in the Taco Seasoning Mix and water and simmer for 5 to 7 minutes, stirring occasionally, until the water has cooked down.
Taco Seasoning Mix (see the following recipe)	
cup water	**3** Pile the corn chips on a large plate. Top with the chicken and capsicum mix. Sprinkle with the cheese.
140 grams baked corn chips	
70 grams grated cheese blend	**4** Place in warm oven until cheese is melted. Top with tomato and avocado and serve warm with salsa (if desired).
1 tomato, diced	
½ avocado, diced	
Fresh salsa (optional)	

Taco Seasoning Mix

Ingredients	Directions
½ teaspoon chilli powder	**1** Mix all ingredients together to form a powder.
¼ teaspoon red pepper flakes	
Pinch of dried oregano	
¼ teaspoon smoked paprika	
1 teaspoon cumin	
¼ teaspoon sea salt	
¼ teaspoon black pepper	

Per serving: Kilojoules 1020/Calories 244 (From Fat 113); Fat 12g (Saturated 5g); Cholesterol 45mg; Sodium 343mg; Carbohydrate 19g (Dietary Fibre 2.5g); Protein 14g; Sugar 2.5g.

Spicy Almonds

Prep time: 10 min • **Cook time:** 1 hour • **Yield:** 12 servings (¼ cup serves)

Ingredients	Directions
⅛ cup brown sugar or ¼ teaspoon of stevia	**1** Preheat oven to 135 degrees Celsius. Coat a large rimmed baking tray with cooking spray.
2 teaspoons ground cumin	**2** Whisk brown sugar or stevia, cumin, paprika, thyme, salt and cayenne in a large bowl.
1 teaspoon hot paprika	
1 teaspoon dried thyme	**3** Whisk egg white and water in a medium bowl until foamy. Add almonds to egg white and stir to coat; pour through a sieve to drain off excess egg white.
1 teaspoon sea salt	
¼ teaspoon cayenne pepper	
1 large egg white	**4** Transfer the almonds to the bowl of spices; stir well to coat. Spread evenly on the prepared baking sheet.
1 tablespoon water	
3 cups raw whole almonds	**5** Bake the almonds for 30 minutes. Mix, reduce the oven temperature to 100 degrees Celsius and bake until the almonds are dry and golden, about 30 minutes more. Allow to cool for about 20 minutes before serving.

Per serving: Kilojoules 607/Calories 145 (From Fat 100); Fat 11.2g (Saturated 0.9g); Cholesterol 0mg; Sodium 199mg; Carbohydrate 7g (Dietary Fibre 3g); Protein 5.4g; Sugar 2.4.

Source: Adapted from recipe by www.ahealthyview.com.

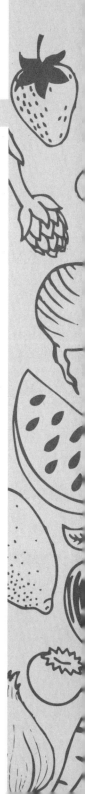

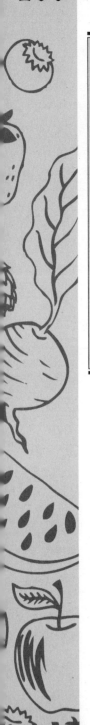

Cooking with stevia

Unbleached stevia may add the sweetness you require during your transition to your low-sugar lifestyle. Sweeteners that come from nature are always better choices than ones that come from a factory or laboratory. Stevia comes from the extract of a herb and has been used as a sweetener for centuries in Japan. It provides 300 times the sweet taste of sugar so you only require small amounts.

Stevia contains zero kilojoules, has little effect on blood glucose levels and contains no fructose. Unlike most artificial sweeteners, stevia is also useful in cooking because the glycosides do not break down in the heat.

To replace sugar with stevia in your cooking, use the following table.

Sugar Amount	Equivalent Unbleached Stevia Powdered Extract	Equivalent Stevia Liquid Concentrate
1 cup	1 teaspoon	1 teaspoon
1 tablespoon	¼ teaspoon	6 to 9 drops
1 teaspoon	A pinch to 1/16 teaspoon	2 to 4 drops

Table reproduced from The Stevia Cookbook by Ray Sahelian and Donna Gates, published by Avery Trade. © Ray Sahelian, M.D. www.raysahelian.com.

Michele recommends travelling with your food. Apples and pears can roll around for days in the car and still be there for when hunger strikes. Even better, a small bag of walnuts or almonds in the glove box can last up to a couple of weeks!

Sweet Potato (Kumara) Pancakes

Prep time: 15 min • **Cook time:** 10–15 min • **Yield:** 4–5 servings (about 10 pancakes)

Ingredients	Directions
¼ **cup almond meal**	**1** Place almond meal, coconut flour, baking powder, sweet potato (or kumara) and pumpkin seeds in a bowl and mix well.
¼ **cup coconut flour**	
½ **teaspoon baking powder**	
100 grams mashed sweet potato or kumara	**2** In a separate bowl, whisk together eggs and coconut milk. Add to dry ingredients and stir well to combine.
¼ **cup pumpkin seeds**	
5 eggs	**3** Heat butter in a fry pan over medium heat and ladle on scoops of the pancake mix. Cook for 2 to 3 minutes each side until golden and cooked through.
¼ **cup coconut milk**	
Coconut oil or butter, for cooking	

Per serving: Kilojoules 1117 /Calories 267(From Fat 160); Fat 17.9g (Saturated 8.9g); Cholesterol 232mg; Sodium 166mg; Carbohydrate 12.7g (Dietary Fibre 4.7g); Protein 12.8g; Sugar 1.5g.

Vary It! Add some corn into the mixture in Step 2 for additional crunch and fibre.

Tip: Sprinkle shredded coconut and some coriander leaves on top before serving.

Source: Adapted from recipe by Thr1ve.me.

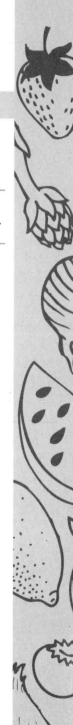

Veggie Burger Patties

Prep time: 10 min • **Cook time:** 10 min • **Yield:** 2 servings

Ingredients	Directions
1 teaspoon extra-virgin olive oil	**1** Preheat the oven to 250 degrees Celsius. Line a flat baking tray with baking paper lightly greased with olive oil.
½ cup cooked chickpeas	
1 teaspoon tomato paste	**2** In a blender, mix the chickpeas, tomato paste, Worcestershire sauce, garlic, salt and pepper.
½ teaspoon Worcestershire sauce	
1 garlic clove, minced	**3** Add the bulgur, onion, parsley, mushrooms and chives. Mix again, only until just blended.
Pinch salt	
Pinch ground black pepper	**4** Flatten the bean mix into two 7-to-10-centimetre patties and bake them on the baking tray for about 5 minutes. Flip each patty and bake for another 5 minutes until slightly browned.
¾ cup cooked bulgur	
1 tablespoon red onion, minced	
1 teaspoon fresh parsley, minced	
1 tablespoon chopped mushrooms of choice	
1 tablespoon chives, minced	

Per serving: Kilojoules 540/Calories 129 (From Fat 65); Fat 7g (Saturated 0.5g); Cholesterol 0mg; Sodium 621mg; Carbohydrate 15g (Dietary Fibre 3.5g); Protein 2.5g; Sugar 0.8g.

Tip: This patty recipe goes well with many different condiments, like mustard or low-sugar chilli sauces. See www.ahealthyview.com.au for some options.

Vary It! Worcestershire sauce contains anchovies, so for a vegan variation, substitute tamari, a wheat-free soy sauce.

Protein-Packed Prawn Salad with Dill Dressing

Prep time: 6 min • **Cook time:** 7 min • **Yield:** 4 servings

Ingredients	Directions
¾ cup white wine 2 bay leaves 1 fresh lemon, sliced 500 grams prawns, peeled and deveined Dill Dressing (see the following recipe) Salt and ground black pepper to taste	**1** In a 2- or 3-litre saucepan, combine the wine, bay leaves and lemon slices. Add water to the pan until it's half full. Bring to a boil over high heat.
	2 Add the fresh prawns and boil for 1 to 2 minutes, until the prawns are pink.
	3 Drain the prawns in a strainer and cool them under cold water. Remove the bay leaves and lemon pieces.
	4 Place the prawns in a clean bowl and add the Dill Dressing. Salt and pepper to taste. Toss well. Refrigerate and serve chilled.

Dill Dressing

3 tablespoons extra-virgin olive oil 3 tablespoons red wine vinegar 1 tablespoon chopped fresh basil 2 tablespoons chopped fresh dill ½ medium onion, chopped 1 teaspoon Dijon mustard	**1** In a medium bowl, whisk together all the ingredients. Optional: Shake vigorously in a shaker cup instead of whisking in a bowl.

Per serving: Kilojoules 933/Calories 223 (From Fat 92); Fat 10.3g (Saturated 1.6g); Cholesterol 157mg; Sodium 709mg; Carbohydrate 4.7g (Dietary Fibre 0.4g); Protein 17.3g; Sugar 1.3g.

Tip: Serve on a bed of fresh, crisp romaine lettuce or on multi-grain crackers.

Guacamole

Prep time: 10 min • **Yield:** 2 servings (¼ cup each)

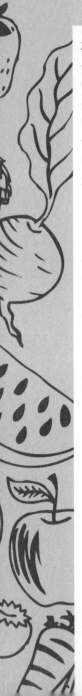

Ingredients	*Directions*
2 avocados, diced	**1** In a medium bowl, mash the avocado with the back of a fork or a potato masher. Mix in the remaining ingredients, except the chips or carrot and celery sticks. Salt and pepper to taste. Serve with baked corn chips or carrot and celery sticks.
½ cup fresh salsa (or finely chopped fresh tomatoes)	
1 tablespoon sour cream or plain Greek yoghurt	
¼ cup chopped fresh coriander	
2 tablespoons fresh lime juice	
1 teaspoon chilli, finely chopped without seeds	
1 Australian (or local) garlic clove, finely minced	
½ cup grated cheese	
Salt and ground black pepper to taste	
Baked corn chips or carrot and celery sticks for serving	

Per serving: Kilojoules 520/Calories 124 (From Fat 88); Fat 9.8g (Saturated 2.7g); Cholesterol 7mg; Sodium 147mg; Carbohydrate 7.4g (Dietary Fibre 4.7g); Protein 3.5g; Sugar 1.1g.

Tip: This guacamole makes a great topping for a baked potato, or side for chicken or fish.

Zucchini Almond Dip

Prep time: 10 min • **Yield:** 2 servings (¼ cup each)

Ingredients	Directions
1 cup of raw almonds, soaked overnight **2 zucchinis, chopped** **2 cloves Australian (or local) garlic** **Juice of ½ a lemon** **¼ teaspoon sea salt** **Ground black pepper to taste**	*1* Puree all ingredients in a food processor until the mixture is smooth. Cut fresh vegetables of your choice for dipping and enjoy this protein-packed dip.

Per serving: Kilojoules 469/Calories 112 (From Fat 75); Fat 9.0g (Saturated 0.71g); Cholesterol 0mg; Sodium 77mg; Carbohydrate 5.9g (Dietary Fibre 2.7g); Protein 4.4g; Sugar 2.0g.

Vary It! To give this dip a Mexican flavour, add ¼ teaspoon of smoked hot paprika and ¼ teaspoon of cayenne pepper to the mixture.

Tip: This makes a great accompaniment to grilled or barbecued fish fillet.

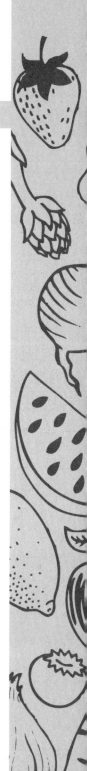

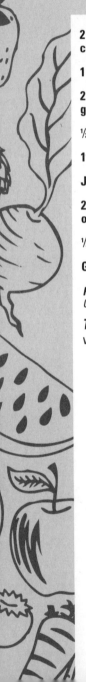

Sweet Potato Hummus Dip

Prep time: 10 min • **Yield:** 2 servings (¼ cup each)

Ingredients	Directions
2 large sweet potatoes, cooked	**1** Place all ingredients in food processor and puree until smooth. Serve with fresh carrot and celery for dipping, or vegetable sticks of your choice.
1 can chickpeas	
2 cloves Australian (or local) garlic	
½ cup tahini	
1 teaspoon ground cumin	
Juice of 1 lemon	
2 tablespoons extra-virgin olive oil	
½ teaspoon sea salt	
Ground black pepper to taste	

Per serving: Kilojoules 2473/Calories 147 (From Fat 40); Fat 4.5g (Saturated 0.65g); Cholesterol 0mg; Sodium 343mg; Carbohydrate 22.6g (Dietary Fibre 4.3g); Protein 4.9g; Sugar 2.4g.

Tip: Use this dip as a sweet potato mash under sliced marinated lamb, beef or chicken and top with a dollop of low-sugar chutney or chilli sauce. Serve with a side of fresh green beans.

Spinach Quiche Muffins

Prep time: 10 min • **Cook time:** 25 min • **Yield:** 8 servings

Ingredients	Directions
1 teaspoon melted butter	**1** Preheat the oven to 175 degrees Celsius. Grease 8 muffin cups with melted butter.
225-gram pack of frozen spinach	
2 eggs	**2** Defrost spinach in the microwave according to the package directions. Squeeze well to drain excess water.
¾ cup grated cheese of choice	
¼ cup diced green capsicum	**3** In a medium bowl, beat the eggs thoroughly. Add the spinach, cheese, capsicum, jalapeño pepper (if using) and mushrooms. Salt and pepper to taste. Mix well and divide evenly into muffin cups.
1 teaspoon minced jalapeño pepper (optional)	
¼ cup diced mushrooms	
Salt and ground black pepper to taste	**4** Bake for 20 minutes, until a toothpick inserted into the centre comes out clean.

Per serving: Kilojoules 326/Calories 78 (From Fat 45); Fat 5g (Saturated 2.5g); Cholesterol 57mg; Sodium 288mg; Carbohydrate 1.5g (Dietary Fibre 0.5g); Protein 5g; Sugar 0.5g.

Vary It! For more protein, add ¼ cup cooked nitrate-free bacon to Step 3.

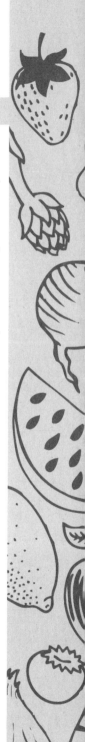

Afternoon Tea Power Smoothie

Prep time: 5 min • **Yield:** 1 serving

Ingredients	Directions
1 scoop of clean whey protein powder	*1* Blend all ingredients for 2 minutes, until smooth. Enjoy!
½ cup frozen raspberries or blueberries	
½ cup coconut water (or A2 milk or almond milk)	
½ cup water	
1 tablespoon chia seeds	
1 teaspoon coconut oil (optional)	

Per serving: Kilojoules 1280/Calories 306 (From Fat 86); Fat 10.1g (Saturated 5.1g); Cholesterol 30mg; Sodium 189mg; Carbohydrate 25.6g (Dietary Fibre 4.3g); Protein 28.3g; Sugar 12.8g.

Vary It! Add ½ teaspoon of cocoa powder or cocoa nibs for a rich chocolate taste without sugar.

Tip: To make a smoothie that has additional protein, add a tablespoon of oats and a tablespoon of your favourite nuts before blending until smooth.

Chapter 17

Sin-Free Desserts

. . . .

In This Chapter

▶ Changing your dessert habits to healthier fare

▶ Upgrading your definition of dessert

. . . .

Dessert. The word inspires excitement in some and dread in others. For some people, finishing every meal by indulging in a sweet decadence has become a lifelong habit. Others eat desserts infrequently but go overboard whenever sugary delights are present. Christmas time can be a nightmare (or a dream come true) for dessert-o-holics, because December tends to bring pavlova, mince pies, biscuits and Christmas sweet treats around every corner.

You're taking steps to reduce or eliminate sugar from your diet, but that doesn't mean that you have to swear off desserts forever. We do recommend that you don't move to desserts until you really have kicked your habit and feel completely in control of your sugar plan. For most people this feeling of control usually comes after around four to six weeks. If you try a sweet dessert too soon, you might find yourself right back on the addictive sugar train.

When you're in complete control of your sugar plan, you can make smart choices to have your dessert and eat it too. This chapter provides some tips to lower the sugar content of the desserts you enjoy. We also offer some ideas to help shift your perception of what dessert can be, so that you can pick healthier alternatives when you decide to indulge in some extra calories.

All the dessert recipes in this chapter are free of processed sugars and artificial sweeteners, but some contain more natural sugar than other recipes in this book. The sugar content in the nutritional analysis section reflects the use of fruit, fruit juice or honey in these recipes.

Whenever possible, you should try to use organic ingredients, hormone-free dairy and pasture-fed eggs in these recipes.

Practising Sugar-Free Satisfaction

Many sugar cravings stem purely from habit — the more sugar (or sweetened foods) you eat, the more you want. When you eat dessert every day, you continue to want dessert every day.

Don't make after-dinner sweets an everyday habit. When you feel like having something sweet after a meal, drink some flavoured mineral water or herbal tea instead, or pick a low-sugar alternative from the following recipes. Reserve the heavy-sugar desserts for very special occasions, if at all. After you start weaning yourself off your daily sugar overload, you'll probably find that those sickly-sweet monstrosities aren't very appealing anymore.

Having something sweet after a meal doesn't mean that you have to cram a thousand kilojoules of apple caramel crumble on top of your evening meal! You love dessert as much as the next person (okay, maybe a lot more), but you have plenty of sensible ways to indulge your sweet tooth without assaulting your pancreas and your innocent liver.

Michele's programs have facilitated hundreds of men, women and teens in their transition to a low-sugar way of life. Her clients consistently say that using naturally sweetened herbal teas saved them from becoming the 'human vacuum' after dinner. So treat yourself to a lovely cup of tea and try one or all of the teas in the following list. If you're feeling exceptionally in need of a sweet hit, don't be afraid to double-bag or even triple-bag your tea for a powerful taste explosion.

- ✔ Black Adder Liquorice tea by Red Seal
- ✔ Bengal Spice or Cinnamon and Apple by Celestial Seasonings
- ✔ Tea Tonic's Warm-Spicy Tea
- ✔ T2's Sencha Sensation and Lemongrass & Ginger

Another strategy healthy people develop is choosing some 'junk' food to incorporate in their diet — but not high-sugar 'junk food'. Most people would perceive potato crisps and popcorn as 'junk food'. However, some chips are oven-baked with olive oil. Popcorn kernels popped on the stove top without hydrogenated trans fats (try coconut oil) are a fun and healthy snack. Real chocolate treats that we have listed in this chapter are not 'junk'. Far from it — they can be highly antioxidant and low in sugar. Welcome to this whole new world!

If you love ice cream, check out David Gillespie's guide to the sugar content in Australian ice-creams at www.howmuchsugar.com. The guide lists ice creams and frozen yoghurts on sale in the average Australian supermarket (many of the same brands are also available in New Zealand) and ranks these products by their sugar content. (***Note:*** A membership payment is required before you can access these guides.)

Insulin-friendly baking tips

To turn high-glycaemic or high-sugar desserts into low-sugar, insulin-friendly treats, try these healthier substitutions with recipes you find outside this book:

- Add whey protein or nuts for extra protein and better blood sugar control.

- Look for ways to add grated carrots, apples or pumpkin in recipes to add more fibre and moisture, while cutting back on the sugar.

- Substitute half the flour called for in a recipe with wholegrain flour like oat flour, brown rice flour or spelt.

- To cut back on calories, replace oil with unsweetened applesauce (using the same measurement), or use only ¾ the amount of oil called for in the recipe.

- Try decreasing the amount of sugar or dried fruit used in a recipe by 25 to 50 per cent of what's called for.

Anzac Biscuits

Prep time: 15 min • **Cook time:** 15 min • **Yield:** 16 biscuits

Ingredients	Directions
¾ cup plain flour	**1** Preheat oven to 175 degrees Celsius. Mix the flour, stevia, coconut, vanilla, cinnamon and oats in a bowl.
⅓ cup stevia granules	
¾ cup shredded coconut	**2** Melt the butter and rice malt syrup together until it bubbles and stir through the baking soda. Add the butter mixture to the dry ingredients in the bowl and stir to combine.
½ teaspoon vanilla powder	
½ teaspoon cinnamon	
¾ cup rolled oats	
100 grams salted butter	**3** Roll heaped teaspoons of the mixture into balls and flatten on a greased tray.
2 tablespoons rice malt syrup	
½ teaspoon baking soda dissolved in 1 tablespoon boiling water	**4** Bake for 15 minutes, or until golden brown.
	5 Remove the biscuits from the oven and cool on a rack to ensure they turn crispy!

Per serving (per cookie): Kilojoules 573/Calories 137 (From Fat 74); Fat 8.3g (Saturated 6g); Cholesterol 15mg; Sodium 92mg; Carbohydrate 12.5g (Dietary Fibre 1.6g); Protein 2.3g; Sugar 2.5g.

Vary It! For a completely gluten-free version, replace the flour with a combo of quinoa and rice flour and replace the oats with ½ cup almond meal.

Source: *Adapted from recipe by Sarah Wilson www.iquitsugar.com.*

Vegan Peanut Butter Biscuits

Prep time: 15 min • **Cook time:** 15 min • **Yield:** 48 biscuits

Ingredients	Directions
2½ cups rolled oats	**1** Preheat the oven to 175 degrees Celsius. Line a baking tray with baking paper.
¼ cup unbleached flour	
⅛ teaspoon cinnamon	**2** In a large mixing bowl, stir together the oats, flour and cinnamon.
2 mashed bananas	
⅓ cup unsweetened peanut butter	**3** In a separate bowl, combine the mashed bananas, peanut butter, soy milk, butter, maple syrup and vanilla. Mix well.
2 tablespoons unsweetened soy or almond milk	
¼ cup melted butter	**4** Combine the banana mixture and the oat mixture and mix well.
2 tablespoons pure maple syrup	
1 teaspoon pure vanilla extract	**5** Drop the batter by teaspoons onto the baking tray.
	6 Bake at 175 degrees for approximately 15 minutes, until firm. Be careful not to let the edges burn.
	7 Remove the biscuits from the oven and transfer them to wire racks to cool.

Per serving: Kilojoules 205/Calories 49 (From Fat 21); Fat 2.5g (Saturated 0.5g); Cholesterol 0mg; Sodium 17mg; Carbohydrate 6g (Dietary Fibre 0.5g); Protein 1g; Sugar 1.3g.

Vary It! Add 2 tablespoons of sesame seeds for extra crunch at Step 4.

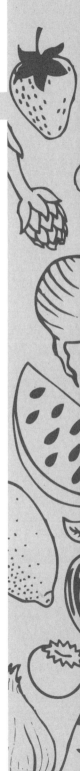

Chocolate Oatmeal Biscuits

Prep time: 10 min • **Cook time:** 12–15 min • **Yield:** 48 biscuits

Ingredients	*Directions*
1 cup wholemeal flour	*1* Preheat the oven to 175 degrees Celsius. Line a baking tray with baking paper.
1 cup rolled oats	
1 cup unsweetened applesauce	*2* In a large mixing bowl, combine all ingredients and mix well.
½ cup sultanas	
½ cup dark chocolate chips or chopped dark chocolate chunks	*3* Drop the batter by teaspoons onto the baking tray.
¼ cup chopped macadamia nuts	*4* Bake for 12 to 15 minutes, until brown.
2 eggs	*5* Remove the cookies from the oven and transfer them to wire racks to cool.
1 teaspoon ground cinnamon	
1 teaspoon baking powder	
½ teaspoon baking soda	
¼ teaspoon nutmeg	
¼ teaspoon allspice	
⅓ cup melted butter	
¼ cup water	
1 teaspoon pure vanilla extract	

Per serving: Kilojoules 217/Calories 52 (From Fat 25); Fat 3g (Saturated 0.5g); Cholesterol 8mg; Sodium 18mg; Carbohydrate 6g (Dietary Fibre 0.5g); Protein 1g; Sugar 2.5g.

Vary It! Instead of sultanas, try dried dates chopped finely for a caramelised sweet taste.

Raw Cocoa Cookies

Prep time: 10 min • **Cook time:** 10–12 min • **Yield:** 48 cookies

Ingredients	Directions
1 cup wholemeal spelt flour **½ cup wholemeal buckwheat flour** **⅓ cup brown sugar (or organic panela)** **⅓ cup oats (quick cook option)** **⅓ cup raw dark cocoa powder** **½ teaspoon baking powder** **⅓ cup chopped macadamia nuts** **⅓ cup sultanas (sulphur-free if possible)** **125g melted butter**	**1** Preheat oven onto 180 degrees Celsius. Line a baking tray with baking paper. **2** Into a large bowl add the spelt flour, buckwheat flour, brown sugar, oats, cocoa powder and baking powder. Whisk to evenly distribute. **3** Stir through nuts and sultanas until well coated with flour mix and evenly distributed. **4** Add melted butter and mix until dry mix comes together. (The mixture will be a bit crumbly but this is fine — it moulds together with a bit of pressure.) **5** Use an ice cream scoop or shaped spoon to place mounds of mix on baking tray. Leave as is or push down for flatter cookies. **6** Bake for 15 minutes, until brown. **7** Remove the cookies from the oven and transfer them to wire racks to cool.

*Per serving (**1 cookie**): Kilojoules 209/Calories 50 (From Fat 25); Fat 2.9g (Saturated 1.5g); Cholesterol 5mg; Sodium 6mg; Carbohydrate 5.6g (Dietary Fibre 0.8g); Protein 0.9g; Sugar 1.6g.*

Source: Adapted from recipe by Cindy Luken www.lukbeautifood.com.

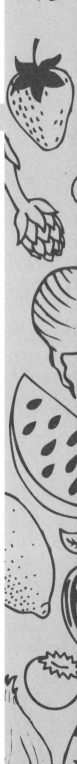

Sugar-Free Brownies

Prep time: 10 min • **Cook time:** 30 min • **Yield:** 12 servings

Ingredients	Directions
1 tablespoon butter (to grease pan)	**1** Preheat the oven to 175 degrees Celsius. Grease the inside of a 22- × 33-centimetre baking pan with butter.
1 cup wholemeal flour	
¼ cup raw dark cocoa powder	**2** In a large mixing bowl, sift together the flour, cocoa powder and baking powder.
½ teaspoon baking powder	
⅔ cup unsweetened apple juice concentrate	**3** Add the apple juice concentrate, melted butter, egg white, walnuts and banana. Mix well.
¼ cup melted butter	
1 egg white	**4** Spread the batter into the prepared pan. Bake at 175 degrees for 30 minutes.
¼ cup chopped walnuts	
1 mashed banana	**5** Remove the brownies from the oven and allow them to cool for a few minutes in the pan before cutting. Serve warm.

Per serving: Kilojoules 582/Calories 139 (From Fat 68); Fat 8g (Saturated 1.5g); Cholesterol 2.5mg; Sodium 18mg; Carbohydrate 17g (Dietary Fibre 2g); Protein 2.5g; Sugar 5.9g.

Coconut Chia Seed Pudding

Prep time: 10 min • **Setting time:** 2 hours • **Yield:** 4 servings

Ingredients	Directions
1½ cups coconut milk 4 tablespoons maple syrup	*1* Whisk coconut milk, maple syrup and extracts until smooth.
1 tablespoon vanilla extract	*2* Stir in chia seeds.
½ teaspoon almond extract ⅓ cup white chia seeds	*3* Divide mixture evenly between four clear glasses and allow to set for two hours.
½ cup blueberries 1 cup coconut shreds	*4* Serve with blueberries and shredded coconut on top.

Per serving: Kilojoules 1987/Calories 475 (From Fat 320); Fat 35.6g (Saturated 28.8g); Cholesterol 0mg; Sodium 25mg; Carbohydrate 32.6g (Dietary Fibre 11.4g); Protein 6.4g; Sugar 15.9g.

Vary It! For a 'Cherry Ripe' pudding, add 2 tablespoons of cocoa powder and substitute the blueberries for raspberries at Step 4.

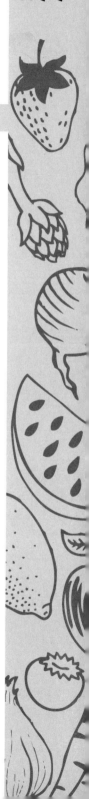

Banana, Coconut and Chia Seed Bread

Prep time: 10 min • **Cook time:** 45–50 min • **Yield:** 1 large loaf (or 12 muffins)

Ingredients	Directions
Melted butter (for greasing)	*1* Preheat the oven to 175 degrees Celsius. Grease the inside of a loaf tin with butter.
3 ripe bananas	
½ cup milk (cow, nut or other)	*2* Place bananas in a large bowl and mash with a potato masher or fork, leaving some chunks.
½ teaspoon baking soda	
2 eggs	*3* Warm the milk in a microwave-safe glass container for 30 seconds.
½ cup melted butter or coconut oil	
1 cup wholemeal buckwheat flour	*4* Carefully add baking soda to the milk and mix until combined. (Beware — the milk will bubble up.) Add the milk mixture to bowl.
1 cup wholemeal spelt flour	
½ cup shredded coconut (fine)	*5* Add eggs and melted butter (or oil) to bowl. Beat with a spoon until well combined.
¾ cup sugar (panela or rapadura)	
1 teaspoon cinnamon	*6* Add all remaining ingredients to bowl. Mix with a spoon until well combined.
2 teaspoons baking powder	
1 teaspoon pure vanilla extract	*7* Pour or spoon mix into tin. Drop tin several times on bench top to spread the mix and knock out any large air bubbles.
	8 Bake for 45 to 50 mins, or until golden brown and a skewer comes out clean. Cool in tin.

Per serving: *Kilojoules 1000/Calories 239 (From Fat 97); Fat 10.8g (Saturated 6.8g); Cholesterol 52mg; Sodium 142mg; Carbohydrate 31.7g (Dietary Fibre 3.5g); Protein 5.0g; Sugar 13.6g.*

Vary It! Top with banana slices and/or sprinkle with rolled oats and chia seeds at Step 7 (before baking).

Source: *Adapted from recipe by Cindy Luken www.lukbeautifood.com.*

Frozen Strawberry Banana Treat

Prep time: 5 min • **Yield:** 1 serving

Ingredients	Directions
¼ cup milk	*1* Place the milk, banana, strawberries, whey protein and ice cubes in a food processor and blend until smooth and whipped.
½ frozen banana	
3 large strawberries	
1 scoop whey protein powder (vanilla or unflavoured)	*2* Core the apple and chop it into ½-inch cubes. Place in serving bowl.
2 ice cubes	
½ apple, any variety	*3* Using a soft spoon or spatula, scrape the frozen treat onto the apple pieces and enjoy.

Per serving: Kilojoules 1150/Calories 275 (From Fat 20); Fat 2g (Saturated 1g); Cholesterol 51mg; Sodium 68mg; Carbohydrate 46g (Dietary Fibre 6g); Protein 22g; Sugar 23g.

Tip: Sprinkle a little fresh chopped mint on top.

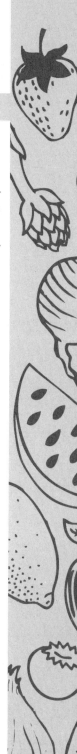

Black Forest Parfait

Prep time: 10 min • **Cook time:** 10 min • **Yield:** 4 servings

Ingredients	Directions
115 grams dark chocolate (70 per cent cocoa), chopped and divided	**1** Chill four parfait glasses in the freezer. Measure 2 tablespoons of the chocolate and set aside.
230 grams frozen or fresh pitted cherries	**2** In a medium saucepan, heat the cherries over medium heat. As the cherries start to heat, simmer until the juice is released, taking care not to let them burn. Remove them from the heat when they are warm and soft.
¼ teaspoon pure vanilla extract	
¼ cup roasted unsalted cashew pieces	**3** To the cherries, stir in the vanilla, cashew pieces, and the remaining chocolate. Allow the mixture to cool slightly but not harden, and then stir in the Stevia powder to taste.
1 teaspoon stevia powder	
4 cups vanilla Greek yoghurt	
	4 Coat each parfait cup with some chocolate cherry mix, and then add alternating layers of yoghurt and chocolate cherry mix.
	5 Top each parfait with the remaining chocolate shavings and serve cold.

Per serving: Kilojoules 2033/Calories 486 (From Fat 167); Fat 19g (Saturated 8g); Cholesterol 1mg; Sodium 122mg; Carbohydrate 52g (Dietary Fibre 4g); Protein 28g; Sugar 46.4g.

Vary It! This parfait is also delicious with blackberries or raspberries instead of cherries. Try it with hazelnuts instead of cashews.

Tip: Use unsweetened/plain Greek yoghurt to lower the sugar content.

Sugar-Free Rhubarb Macaroon Slice

Prep time: 20 min • **Cook time:** 25–30 min • **Yield:** 12 servings

Ingredients	Directions
200 grams rhubarb, cut into 1-centimetre slices	*1* Preheat the oven to 180 degrees Celsius and line a 25- × 15-centimetre baking tray with baking paper.
1 teaspoon ground cinnamon	
¼ teaspoon pure, ground vanilla bean	*2* For the filling, place the rhubarb, ground cinnamon and vanilla, along with a couple of tablespoons of water into a small saucepan. Bring the mixture to boil and then let simmer. Cook the mixture until quite thick, stirring occasionally. Set aside to cool.
100 grams quinoa flakes	
50 grams coconut flakes (no sugar added)	
50 grams rolled oats	*3* While the filling is cooking, make the base. Place the quinoa flakes, coconut flakes, oats and cacao into a food processor. Grind the ingredients into a fine(ish) mixture, then add the coconut oil and grind until the mixture comes together. Beat in the egg whites. Spoon the mixture into the baking tray and, using your hands, spread onto the baking sheet to make a 1- to 2-centimetre thick base.
1 tablespoon raw pure cacao nibs (or cocoa powder)	
80 grams virgin coconut oil	
2 large egg whites (for base)	
3 large egg whites (for top)	*4* For the topping, beat the egg whites in a clean bowl until thick. Carefully fold in the coconut.
50 grams fine desiccated coconut (no sugar added)	
	5 Spread the rhubarb filling on the base into a thin layer. Spread the coconut 'meringue' on top.
	6 Bake at 180 degrees for 25 to 30 minutes, until golden on top. Let cool completely before cutting.

Per serving: Kilojoules 707/Calories 169 (From Fat 108); Fat 12.1g (Saturated 10.7g); Cholesterol 0mg; Sodium 29mg; Carbohydrate 11.9g (Dietary Fibre 3.2g); Protein 4.3g; Sugar 1.0g.

Vary It! To make this gluten-free, use uncontaminated oats, or simply replace the oats with more quinoa flakes.

Source: Adapted from recipe by www.scandifoodie.blogspot.com.au.

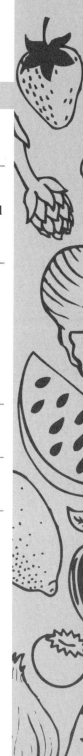

Part V
The Part of Tens

web extras

Find tips to enhance your sleep, which helps with weight loss and anti-ageing, at www.dummies.com/extras/beatingsugaraddictionau.

In this part . . .

- ✔ Figure out which sugar-laden and unhealthy foods to leave at the store when food shopping.

- ✔ Outwit your sugar cravings with smart habits like drinking more water and choosing healthy snacks.

Chapter 18

Ten Surprising Foods to Leave at the Supermarket

*U*nless you grow your own vegetables and raise your own livestock, the supermarket is where you make primary food decisions for you and your family. Though most people recognise the junk-food quality of obvious high-sugar foods like confectionery, lollies and ice-cream, many unhealthy items are available in food shops that you may erroneously think of as healthier alternatives. This chapter explains ten of these foods that, on the surface, may appear to be healthy choices, but in reality are not. When you come across these foods while shopping, keep walking!

If you're interested in making a complete dietary overhaul to all-natural foods, check out *Detox Diets For Dummies* by Gerald Don Wootan and Matthew Brittain Phillips (Wiley) and think about making an appointment with a nutritionist to discuss your detox and cleanse plan. See www.ahealthyview.com.au for a local wholefood cleanse program.

Diet Soft Drinks

Diet soft drinks are sugar-free and calorie-free, so they must be a healthier alternative to sugared soft drinks, right? Wrong.

Diet drinks are artificially sweetened with aspartame (NutraSweet) or other artificial sweeteners, a chemical that causes brain damage and can increase appetite. The type of caramel colouring used in many diet sodas may be a carcinogen. The phosphoric acid in sodas leeches calcium out of your bones, contributing to poor bone density. Stay away from soft drinks of all types, both sugared and zero-calorie!

Even with the harmful ingredients, some people think that diet soft drinks can help them in their transition to a low-sugar way of life. In our experience, this is not the case for the majority of our clients. The sweet taste of artificial sweeteners creates messages that turn on your appetite — especially your appetite for more sweets.

If you like the bubbles of soft drinks, drink sparkling mineral water instead. You can flavour it with fresh lemon or lime.

If the fizz of mineral water is too fast a transition for you (but you have at least given it a go), try adding stevia powder instead of sugar or chemical sweeteners to your beverages. *Stevia* is a natural, plant-based sweetener that has virtually no calories and doesn't carry the health risks that artificial sweeteners do. Over time you can gradually decrease the amount of stevia powder that you put in your water, coffee or tea, until you don't feel like you need any added flavouring any more.

Frozen Meals

'Healthy' frozen meals became popular in the 1980s, as food manufacturers tried to capitalise on consumers' desire for healthier alternatives to TV dinners. Because today's brands of health-conscious meals are low in fat and calories, many dieters believe that they're making a smart decision by eating these handy products. A quick look at the ingredients list shows that this isn't the case.

For example, we selected a glazed chicken meal from the most popular line of 'healthy' frozen foods at the supermarket. It's a low-calorie dinner and you could call it 'lean', but it sure isn't healthy. Here are some of the issues with the ingredients in this frozen meal:

- ✔ The chicken tenderloins undoubtedly come from barn hens, loaded with antibiotics and chemicals (refer to Chapter 6).

- ✔ The chicken is coated with high-fructose corn syrup, several preservatives, salt and artificial colour.

- ✔ The rice accompanying the chicken is blanched, enriched rice, meaning that all the nutrients have been stripped away, leaving just the carbohydrate shell. It also contains partially hydrogenated oil (trans fats), sugar, maltodextrin (more sugar) and caramel colouring.

- ✔ The vegetables are green beans with 'natural flavours' (which can be anything, often a code for monosodium glutamate, or MSG) and wheat grain.

To top off the harmful ingredients, you're supposed to microwave the whole meal in the accompanying plastic tray. When plastics are heated, toxic chemicals leak out. These are known as *BPA*, or bisphenol A, which may be carcinogenic and create endocrine disruption. The National Institute of Environmental Health Sciences in the United States advises against microwaving polycarbonate plastics or putting them in the dishwasher, because the plastic may break down over time and allow BPA to leach into foods. Heat your food in glass containers instead or on the stovetop!

Frozen dinners don't really save much time — it doesn't take long to chop up some organic chicken and vegetables and make a stir-fry with fresh ingredients that you control. Taking a few minutes to throw together a homemade meal like this ensures that you eat healthy ingredients and avoid dangerous chemicals. In other words, it's like creating and nurturing your own 'wellness insurance'.

Bacon and Processed Meats

Pizza with pepperoni and sausage on a Friday night, a bacon and egg roll at the football on Saturday for brekkie, a ham roll for lunch, and pasta with chorizo for dinner? This is not an uncommon weekend menu for many Australians and New Zealanders. Bacon and processed meats have experienced a rise in popularity during the latest resurgence of high-protein diets; however, many health experts have concerns. The World Cancer Research Fund estimates about 10 per cent of bowel cancer is linked to processed meat.

Conventional bacon, sausages and processed meats are made from barn pigs and are usually loaded with nitrates and other preservatives, sugars, artificial smoke flavouring, chemical colouring and MSG. Most supermarket bacon is primarily fat and chemicals.

If you really love bacon and processed meats, find a butcher who uses free-range goods that are nitrate-free.

Canned Soups

A piping hot bowl of chicken soup or chilli sounds like a healthy meal. Even though meat and vegetables are the primary ingredients, canned soup typically contains processed meats, too much salt, sugar, MSG and preservatives.

Many companies still use cans with *bisphenol-A* (BPA) in the lining. BPA is a chemical that acts as an artificial oestrogen and has been linked to several negative health consequences.

If you don't want to make your own soup, look for brands that are made from organic ingredients, without chemical additives, and that are sold in BPA-free containers or pouches. Food manufacturers are getting wise to healthier options, you just have to seek them out.

Genetically Modified Foods

In the 1990s, food manufacturers began using plants that had gone through a process of genetic engineering — inserting genes from other plants, animals or bacteria to alter the crop's genome. Foods that have been genetically modified — often referred to as *GM foods* or *GMOs* (genetically modified organisms) — have caused concern among some members of the scientific community for possible human and environmental health risks, such as infertility, organ damage and immune system problems.

In 1988, more than 60 countries voted unanimously against the use of GMOs in food production and agriculture because the scientific consensus was that unacceptable risks were involved: threats to human health, a negative and irreversible environmental impact, and incompatibility with sustainable agriculture practices. According to Food Standards Australia and New Zealand, GM foods, ingredients, additives or processing aids that contain novel DNA or protein must be labelled with the words 'genetically modified'.

The main sources of GM foods are canola and cotton, but other GM foods come from imported foods and imported GM foods are also used as ingredients in packaged foods sold in Australia and New Zealand. Sadly, where GM ingredients are highly refined, they do not require labelling. For example, soy flour in bread may have come from imported GM soybeans.

No-one knows for certain what harm these products will end up causing to people's bodies and the environment. Our guess is that certain modifications are probably harmless, but some of them are certainly not. Unfortunately, only time will tell. In the meantime, we advise you to stay away from genetically engineered food products whenever possible. By law, food labelled '100 per cent organic' can't contain genetically modified ingredients, so look for that label when shopping.

Microwave Popcorn

You may consider popcorn to be a low-calorie, high-fibre snack, but microwave popcorn isn't a healthy choice. When microwaved, popcorn bags may leak *perfluorooctanoic acid* (PFOA) and other plastic residues into your food. PFOA has been linked to infertility, thyroid disease and a host of other endocrine disorders. Manufacturing giant Dupont has just agreed to not use PFOAs in the manufacturing of their cookware due to the potential health concerns.

Aside from the packaging, commercial microwave popcorn typically contains harmful trans fats, preservatives, artificial colours, sugar, chemical sweeteners and other 'flavour enhancers' like MSG. Read the ingredients once and you'll never touch a bag again.

To avoid dangerous chemicals, pop your own popcorn at home with an air popper or on the stove with some butter or coconut oil and top with herbs and/or sea salt.

Fruit Juice and Juice Drinks

Even though fruit juice is loaded with vitamins and antioxidants, even 100 per cent juice contains too much sugar to be a good choice for those who are trying to limit their sugar intake. Excess fructose (fruit sugar) may cause body fat accumulation, increased appetite, liver disease, and elevated cholesterol and triglycerides. Consult Chapter 3 for more information about fructose.

Eat your fruit whole and fresh. It contains fibre and nutrients and doesn't spike your insulin the way pure juice does. Juice drinks, such as juice cocktails or juice boxes (poppers) for kids, are often only 10 to 20 per cent fruit juice, with the rest of the ingredients being high-fructose corn syrup and other sweeteners, artificial colours and preservatives.

A 250-millilitre bottle of orange juice has approximately 25 grams of sugar. You (or your kids) likely find drinking this amount of juice — and consuming that amount of sugar — easy. However, it would not be so easy to eat the four to five fresh oranges that made that 250-millilitre bottle!

Rice Cakes

Any all-carbohydrate snack — especially if it's made of processed, enriched grains — causes an insulin spike followed by a blood sugar crash several hours later. Rice cakes, some 'healthy' muesli bars and other all-carb snacks aren't good choices for sugar addicts because the lack of protein keeps them on the blood sugar roller-coaster and stimulates cravings.

Have a rice cake (wholegrain, not enriched) topped with peanut butter or any nut butter, or cheese adds fat and protein to mitigate the insulin response and keep your blood sugar levels more stable.

Protein Bars

Most of the protein bars found on the shelves of grocery stores and health food stores are laden with sugars, syrups, preservatives and *fractionated oils* (oils that are processed to become more saturated than they are naturally) — they're basically junk food with added protein.

Not all protein snack bars are loaded with chemicals. Visit www.ahealthyview.com.au for current recommendations for healthy, all-natural snack bars, or to view recipes on how to make your own.

Peanut Butter

Though natural peanut butter is a good source of healthy fats and protein, commercial brands are often made with hydrogenated oils (trans fats) to keep the oil from separating to the top of the jar. Commercial brands also add sugar and sometimes other additives like preservatives and flavourings.

Stick with organic, natural peanut butter. The ingredients should have no more than two items: peanuts and (maybe) salt. Refrigerate natural peanut butter after opening and stirring, or leave the container upside down so the oil mixes through as it moves back to the 'top'.

Chapter 19

Ten Ways to Outwit Your Cravings

In This Chapter

▶ Getting enough water, vegetables, exercise and sleep

▶ Being mindful and choosing healthy alternative activities to eating

S ugar is everywhere, and resisting the urge to overindulge may seem difficult — but can become easy with the tips in this chapter. Stress, poor nutrition, dehydration and lack of sleep can all drive you to grab whatever sugar-laden food is handy. Building good habits — lifelong habits — is an essential task for staying off sugar. In this chapter, we lay out ten healthy habits and lifestyle changes that help minimise both the number and the intensity of any sugar cravings you may experience. If you make these principles part of how you live every day, soon your life as a sugar-free, productive, vibrant person will be your norm.

Eat Small Amounts of Food Every Three to Four Hours

'When you skip, you dip' is a saying that Michele likes to get her clients to think about. Even if you're not hungry at morning tea and afternoon tea, we suggest you have something small and protein-packed, especially for the first six weeks of this transition. Low blood sugar can fire up cravings for high-sugar food. When blood sugar plummets, your energy drops and your brain has trouble focusing, making turning to sugar for a quick pick-me-up all too easy. Eating every three or four hours throughout the day helps keep your blood sugar levels more even and the sugar cravings at bay. You also won't be as hungry at night, so resisting late-night sweet fixes is easier. (If one sure way exists to mess up your blood sugar and gain weight, it's eating sweets late at night. Late night food cheats are often those who haven't properly fed themselves throughout the day.)

Every time you eat, try to combine a *protein* and a *plant* (refer to Chapter 5).

Drink Enough Water throughout the Day

Don't confuse hunger for thirst. Even a small amount of dehydration can trigger the hypothalamus to activate the hunger and thirst centres. As we discuss in Chapter 5, drinking enough water — at least 1.5 to 2 litres per day — is one of the easiest ways to keep sugar cravings in check. Doing so also cuts down on your desire for other, less healthy beverages.

Downing a glass of room temperature water with a squeeze of lemon is one of the first things you should do when a sugar craving strikes. Michele even encourages all her clients to drink one full glass of water upon rising, even before going to the toilet! (Refer to Chapter 9 for more on dealing with sugar cravings.)

Take Your Vitamins

A deficiency of one or more important vitamins or minerals can cause your brain to turn on the craving centre in an attempt to take in more nutrients. A smart nutrition supplementation program ensures that you have all the vital nutrients you need to stay healthy, vibrant and sugar-free.

Flip to Chapter 5 for an introduction to helpful nutrition supplements, and visit www.ahealthyview.com.au for a list of recommended brands.

Stay Mindful

To stay on track with a sensible nutrition plan, and to avoid eating according to unconscious cues and temptations, you must remain mindful about when you eat, what you choose, and how much you consume. Before you begin eating, set out your portion so you're not eating from bags or serving dishes. Avoid eating mindlessly in front of the television. Chew thoroughly, and pay careful attention to the whole experience of eating. What does your food really taste and smell like? In between every bite, assess whether you've had enough to eat so that you're not using external cues like an empty plate to tell you when it's time to stop. Turn to Chapter 8 for a more in-depth discussion of mindful eating.

Consider learning some basic meditation techniques. They'll help you stay more centred and present throughout your whole day and help make mindful eating second nature. Check out *Meditation For Dummies* by Stephan Bodian (published by Wiley), which includes a CD with guided meditations.

Eat Lots of Vegetables Every Day

Most of your carbohydrates should come from vegetables. Think about eating a variety of colourful vegetables throughout the day for the greatest amount of phytonutrients. Though whole grains contain some quality nutrients, they're also higher in calories and typically have a higher glycaemic load than vegetables. Fibrous vegetables like broccoli, bok choy and greens are low in calories and high in nutrients and fibre, so they should make up the bulk of your carbohydrate intake.

When it comes to complete nutrition, variety is key. Refer to the fruit and vegetable colour chart (which groups fruits and vegetables according to colour) in Chapter 6, and regularly try to eat a wide spectrum of vegetables and fruits of various colours. Think about eating a rainbow of colour every day.

Exercise

Regular exercise unquestionably helps you lose weight, improves your insulin sensitivity, and increases your metabolism. Exercise can also make your skin radiant because it increases your blood flow. Additionally, it can help you feel great and give you something to do besides eat. If you're not comfortable at a gym, you can start doing some workouts at home or begin a modest walking program four or five days per week.

Refer to Chapter 12 for an overview of exercise basics.

Choose a Positive Substitute Behaviour When a Craving Strikes

Whenever a sugar craving strikes, making a conscious decision to do something other than eat sugar is a healthy and empowering alternative. Positive activities like exercising, learning, creating something new, connecting with friends and helping other people give you an alternative activity to gobbling down the sweet stuff, and add more empowerment to your life. Experiment with some of the positive substitute activities in Chapter 9 and see what works for you.

Avoid Boredom

Some people eat when they're bored, but mindless or reactive eating is never a good idea, especially if the convenient snacks lying around are the high-sugar or high-carb type. If your brain is craving some stimulation, give it something better to do than catatonic chewing! Keep your mind active with crossword or Sudoku puzzles, reading, creative writing or other brain-nourishing tasks. Getting up and doing something also helps — take a walk or practise a musical instrument to replace mindless eating and to limit your consumption of extra empty calories.

If you're the type who gets bored easily, make a 'go to' list of brain-stimulating activities, or a list of 'things that must eventually get done'. The next time boredom strikes, get your brain back in gear by picking an activity from your list.

Get Enough Sleep

Lack of sleep has been proven to contribute to increases in both body fat and appetite. Sleep deprivation also impairs problem solving, alertness, concentration, reasoning and attention (that's why it's one of the leading causes of car accidents and workplace injuries). When you don't sleep well, you feel tired and crave sugar to artificially generate energy. Try to get at least seven hours of solid sleep each night.

Consider a magnesium or melatonin supplement before bed (*melatonin* is a hormone that helps regulate sleep patterns and some current research claims that it may offer protection against cancer), or try a cup of valerian or chamomile tea. Speak to a nutritionist or health practitioner before you begin any supplement.

Don't Let Triggers Set You Off

It's easy to fall into the trap of reactive behaviour, including making poor food choices when you feel stressed. Much of the anxiety and stress people experience is caused purely by their imagination about what's happening or what they're afraid will happen. Being aware of the truth of the present situation (instead of making up stories in your head and reacting to them) is crucial to maintaining healthy eating habits and a healthy overall emotional state.

The key to overcoming stress eating (and reactive behaviour in general) is to become very clear about what you really want. When you experience an emotional trigger, force yourself to do a quick reality check to determine what you really need. For example, if you feel stressed and overwhelmed, what you really want is peacefulness and personal power, not sugar. If you're unhappy with the behaviour of your spouse, what you probably need is to feel reassured and reconnected with your partner — sugar can't give you that. And if you're exhausted, sleep is the answer, not sugar.

The simple steps to stop stress eating are:

1. **Recognise when you've been triggered.**

2. **Stop and figure out what you really need and if you have eaten properly in the previous meal.**

3. **Make a conscious — not reactive — decision.**

We invite you to really dig into Chapter 9 to get a more thorough understanding of emotional triggers and advice on how to stop the cycle of reactive behaviour and stress eating. It's one of the most life-changing chapters in this book!

Index

• R •

• S •

About the Authors

Michele Chevalley Hedge is the owner and founder of A Healthy View and works as a nutritionist, health writer and presenter in Sydney, Australia. When it comes to increasing vitality, clearing brain fog, balancing moods, preventing disease, and keeping yourself in optimum mental and physical condition, Michele believes that good nutrition is proving to be key. Michele is often introduced as the 'modern-day nutritionist' who loves to eat and cook, and believes 'extremes' do not work — real food does.

Dan DeFigio is the owner and director of Basics and Beyond fitness & nutrition and works as a nutrition counsellor, rehabilitative exercise specialist and author in Nashville, Tennessee. Over his 20-year career, Dan has appeared on *Dr. Phil* and in *SELF* magazine, *MD News* and a slew of other media outlets. In addition to teaching exercise and nutrition, Dan is a former mixed martial arts fighter, and some say he is quite a piano player.

Dedication

From Michele: *Beating Sugar Addiction For Dummies* is dedicated to you, a wellness seeker. And to all the millions of people who are incredibly wise for seeking preventative health and wellness through a foundation of nutritious food. No greater gift exists than a healthy mind and body, and these begin with how you feed yourself. You may have struggled your entire life with sugar addictions, poor food choices and self-sabotage — now you are on your way. May this book and the current wave of 'nutritional transformation' catch you and lead you to a balanced and empowered physical, mental and emotional body.

From Dan: This book is dedicated to the millions of people who struggle with achieving a healthy lifestyle — frustrated dieters, sugar addicts, diabetics, desk jockeys, frenzied soccer mums and all those who can't seem to escape the whirlwind of stress and anxiety in their lives. May this book lead you toward empowerment, peace and success.

This book is also dedicated to the wellness professionals who serve these millions — the doctors, nutritionists, therapists, fitness trainers, nurses, chiropractors, yoga teachers and health coaches who lead the way for so many who desire to be healthier. If you've changed one life, you've made a difference.

Authors' Acknowledgements

From Michele: First and foremost, I want to express my deepest gratitude to Gabrielle, Jacob, Holly and to Steven for your support of my relentless passion for and deep trust in good nutrition. Without your support, A Healthy View and Cleanse & Nourish Retreats (www.ahealthyview.com.au) would not have been born. You have allowed me the education, experiences and joy of guiding people to nutritional wellness and simply feeling good about themselves.

The award for 'I couldn't have done it without you' goes to Susan Searle, a firm believer in me, and my backbone in writing this book. Thanks for your outstanding editing skills, attention to detail and all-round 'fabulousness'.

A special thank you to the dedicated team at John Wiley & Sons, especially to Clare Dowdell, for seeking me out for this project, and to Dani Karvess, project editor, and Charlotte Duff, copy editor, for your time and patience in creating a very readable and enticing *For Dummies* book.

Thanks also to my patients, cleansers, readers, dearest friends and most amazing colleagues — I would be remiss not to mention you all. I am full of big love for your nourishment of my soul. I am also reminded daily that I get to work with amazing people who are not only incredibly intelligent practitioners but also generous of heart, which makes them outstanding mentors. Thank you Lara Grinevitch, Kira Sutherland, Michelle Markwick, Rhoslyn Humphrey, Terri Boyce and Jane Sidd.

Finally, I owe a great deal to Rene and Catherine Chevalley. I am thankful to Rene, my dad, for sharing his love of fine, nutritious food even when we had to grow it in our own greenhouse. I am blessed by Catherine, my mum, for encouraging me to deeply believe that 'yes, food is love'.

From Dan: Thank you to the thousands of clients of Basics and Beyond fitness & nutrition (www.gettingfit.com) for your enthusiasm and dedication to wellness. Without your desire to improve yourselves, my team and I wouldn't have our fulfilling careers, and I wouldn't have had the experiences leading me to write this book.

I'd also like to extend special thanks to the staff at John Wiley & Sons, especially Tracy Boggier for seeking me out for this project and Elizabeth Rea, Todd Lothery, Danielle Voirol and Susan P. Watson for turning my nerdy ramblings into a readable *For Dummies* book.

I want to thank two giants in the nutrition science field: Dr Michael Colgan (http://colganinstitute.com) and Dr Thomas Incledon (www.humanhealthspecialists.com). The two of you are an inspiration to the nutrition science field, and we as nutrition professionals can't thank you enough for your enormous contributions to nutrition research and awareness.

Special thanks go out to Susan Carter B.P.E. at the Vanderbilt Center for Integrative Health (www.vcih.org) for your unbelievable passion and enthusiasm for this project. The world could use more people like you!

I owe a great deal to Dr Mitch Johnson at the Center for Spiritual Living Nashville (www.cslnashville.org) and to Anke Nowicki (http://ankenowicki.com) for assisting my journey of self-inquiry and personal growth. Without the two of you, I couldn't be where I am today, and for that you have my eternal gratitude.

Publisher's Acknowledgements

We're proud of this book; please send us your comments through our online registration form located at dummies.custhelp.com.

Some of the people who helped bring this book to market include the following:

Acquisitions, Editorial and Media Development

Project Editor: Charlotte Duff

Acquisitions Editor: Clare Dowdell

Editorial Manager: Dani Karvess

Production

Graphics: diacriTech

Technical Reviewer: Kira Sutherland

Recipe Tester: Emily Nolan

Nutritional Analyst: Nutritionist Rachelle LaCroix Mallik

Proofreader: Kerry Laundon

Indexer: Don Jordan, Antipodes Indexing

The author and publisher would like to thank the following copyright holders, organisations and individuals for their permission to reproduce copyright material in this book:

- **Cover image:** © Hugh Threlfall/Getting Images

- **Page 110 to 111:** List of top 20 Australian foods with the most pesticide detections (2000 to 2011) © Friends of the Earth.

- **Page 111 to 112:** List of top 20 NZ foods with the most pesticide residues © Alison White Safe Food Campaign www.safefood.org.nz.

- **Pages 188 to 201 (Chapter 12):** Photographs © Shannon Fontaine Photography.

Every effort has been made to trace the ownership of copyright material. Information that enables the publisher to rectify any error or omission in subsequent editions is welcome. In such cases, please contact the Legal Services section of John Wiley & Sons Australia, Ltd.

Notes

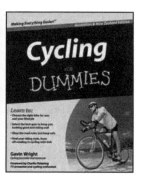
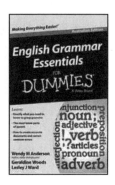
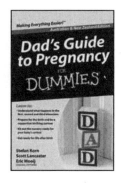
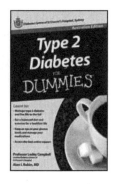

Fitness

Aussie Rules For Dummies,
2nd Edition
978-0-7314-0595-4

Cycling For Dummies,
Australian &
New Zealand Edition
978-0-7303-7664-4

Fishing For Dummies,
2nd Australian &
New Zealand Edition
978-1-74216-984-2

Fitness For Dummies,
Australian &
New Zealand Edition
978-1-74031-009-3

Pilates For Dummies,
Australian Edition
978-1-74031-074-1

Rugby Union For Dummies,
2nd Australian &
New Zealand Edition
978-0-7303-7656-9

Weight Training
For Dummies
2nd Edition
978-0-7303-7660-6

Weight Training
For Dummies,
Australian &
New Zealand Edition
978-1-74031-044-4

Yoga For Dummies,
Australian &
New Zealand Edition
978-1-74031-059-8

History

Australian History
For Dummies
978-1-74216-999-6

Australian Politics
For Dummies
978-1-74216-982-8

Kokoda For Dummies,
Australian Edition
978-0-7303-7699-6

Tracing Your Family History
Online For Dummies,
Australian Edition
978-1-74031-071-0

Health & Health Care

Breast Cancer For Dummies,
Australian Edition
978-1-74031-143-4

Dad's Guide to Pregnancy
For Dummies, Australian
& New Zealand Edition
978-0-7303-7735-1

Food & Nutrition
For Dummies,
Australian &
New Zealand Edition
978-0-7314-0596-1

IVF & Beyond For Dummies,
Australian Edition
978-1-74216-946-0

Kids' Food Allergies
For Dummies, Australian
& New Zealand Edition
978-1-74246-844-0

Living Gluten-free
For Dummies,
Australian Edition
978-0-7314-0760-6

Menopause For Dummies,
Australian Edition
978-1-74031-140-3

Pregnancy For Dummies,
3rd Australian &
New Zealand Edition
978-0-7303-7739-9

Type 2 Diabetes
For Dummies,
Australian Edition
978-1-118-30362-7

Reference

English Grammar
For Dummies,
2nd Australian Edition
978-1-118-49327-4

English Grammar Essentials
For Dummies,
Australian Edition
978-1-118-49331-1

Freelancing for Australians
For Dummies
978-0-7314-0762-0

Passing Exams For Dummies
978-1-7421-6925-5

Writing Essays For Dummies
978-0-470-74290-7

Order today! Contact your Wiley sales representative.

ℯ Available in print and e-book formats.

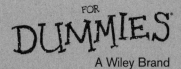

A Wiley Brand

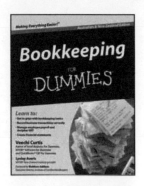
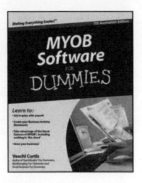
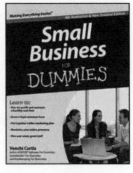
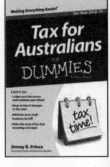